Abyssal Heights

Michael Yanuck MD PhD

DEDICATION

For Dvora & Abba Caspi, Marietta Karpe,
John, Jane, Steve, Phalla, Marina & Conan Dixon,
Barbara, Cliff & Hillary Johnson, Hanne D'Ortiz,
Marge and David Schneider,
and especially Sara.

Names of people and places have been changed and most of the characters represent composites of more than one person. Although not always presented in the order they occurred, the events of this story are otherwise based on real events.

A novel is never anything but a philosophy put into images.
~ Albert Camus

To: Michael Kadima, MD

From: Bradley Lang, MD

Re: Notice of Performance Deficiency

cc: Personnel file

Since you began work at FQHC, your work performance has not meet FQHC standards and this has resulted in a number of performance deficiencies including substandard clinical management for potentially life-threatening medical concerns by prescribing medication for a patient to which she had a documented allergy to medication in a similar class.

In reviewing your charts over the past 9 months we have noted a similar type of performance deficiency: Patient prescribed azithromycin (a macrolide) for respiratory infection. It was prescribed despite the documentation of an allergy to erythromycin (also a macrolide).

Your work performance does not meet FQHC standards and this has resulted in a number of patient and staff complaints. Please note that your contract specifies the following: 'FQHC may immediately terminate your employment if you fail or refuse to perform your duties to FQHC's general satisfaction, or otherwise breach any provision of the contract.'

Specific remediation includes achieving 100% compliance with FQHC's expectation for documentation in history of present illness, physical examination, assessment and treatment section in the chart.

Please consider this letter of reprimand to be formal notice of your performance deficiencies. You have 30 days to remedy these issues...

CHAPTER ONE

Arriving at FQHC, Inc. headquarters, the Chief Executive Officer was leading a meeting of the medical staff.

"Federally Qualified Health Centers, Inc. is committed to being the most transparent healthcare organization in the country," he said. "We are carrying out that commitment because the American people have a right to know what organizations like ours is doing to provide them improved care."

"Most important, customer satisfaction is job one," he continued. "Docs, your job is simple; client comes to you with a problem, you give them a pill. Easy. That's what doctors are for. You're in the drug-delivery business."

He smiled and those in attendance laughed.

"Let's face it," the CEO asserted. "Patients don't really need to talk — that's not going to cure them. What's going to help them are drugs. And at FQHC, we want to make it as easy for the client as possible. That's why we have our own pharmacy downstairs. We're here to provide our customers with all their one-stop shopping needs."

Most of the physicians were nodding, though I noticed one among them who stood hunched in the back of the room, his long white coat pulled tight around his long, thin frame, and his expression doubtful, as he surveyed those in attendance.

"Now, I have the pleasure of introducing the newest physician to join our firm," the CEO announced. "Dr. Michael Kadima acquired his medical training at the Midland College of Medicine. For a long time he did cancer research; but after an injury and learning what it was to be a patient himself, he's returned to medicine and even enlisted in the National Health Service Corps. Let's welcome him to

FQHC."

The physicians clapped respectfully, and then stepped forward to shake my hand. The last of them was the doubtful-looking one who had been standing in the back.

"Brad Lang," he said. "Family practice. Sounds like you've done a lot, Mike. How did you wind up in a place like this?"

The declining health of my fiancée's grandmother, I said. She and the family live nearby. In fact, the grandmother had actually worked in this building for thirty years as a children's social worker before FQHC came to occupy the site.

Brad nodded.

"Why'd you sign up for the NHSC?" he asked. "Did you owe a couple hundred thousand in loans that they paid off?"

I shook my head.

No, I said. I only had $2,000 worth of loans left when I applied.

"$2,000?!" he responded. "You could have made that in a couple of nights moonlighting at Abyssal Heights General. That's where we send most of our patients. Their ER is always short-staffed. They would have taken you in a heartbeat. You didn't have to sign up for the NHSC."

I did it because I believe in what the NHSC stands for, I said. Providing care for those most in need.

"So, you're a crusader," he said. "Well, you sure did find yourself a good mud pile to work in…"

CHAPTER TWO

Lang looked about.

"Oh, well," he continued. "I guess it could have been worse. You could've wound up at an Indian Reservation."

Looking away I decided to withhold comment.

Lang sighed.

"I remember my first day at FQHC," he said. "I was driving to work and a woman pulled me over on the road. She said that she'd been diagnosed with cancer, and came here from another state to continue her chemotherapy, 'cause she couldn't afford the treatment there. But she only had $500 when she left, but had spent all that, and now needed money for the Super 8 just up the road. I said, 'OK, I'll help you with the money for the motel room.' But when I called the Super 8, there was no listing of her name or that she'd ever been there.

"And that's the problem with this population, especially with patients like the ones who show up here. They'll take advantage of you, and squeeze you for everything you've got. It will take everything you have to try to pull these people up. And I don't know how much it will leave you for anything else."

Lang walked me to my desk, located in the same office as his.

"You'll get to know how it works here," he said. "Administration runs the show. When they say jump, you just better hope you clear the bar."

But like the name says, I responded, this is a 'Federally Qualified Health Center.' It's overseen by the government.

"Yeah, that's what I thought, too," he responded. "But FQHC is a corporation. It gets about half a million for being a FQHC, but after that, as long as the clinic's pushing a patient through every fifteen minutes and hitting the right performance numbers, the feds don't care what else goes on."

"So, take some advice," he concluded. "Do what you're told and don't cross Administration."

"You won't have to worry about Administration," came a female voice from behind.

Looking over my shoulder, the Clinical Director, Dr. Jessica Sullivan, strode confidently towards us.

"Not as long as I'm here," she added.

Lang looked cross.

"We'll see," he responded.

He moved off.

"Hey, Brad, wait," she called after him.

Catching up with him, I watched as the two spoke in the hallway – Jessica pleading, as Lang stood arms folded, chest caved, head bent and gaze directed downwards…

CHAPTER THREE

Jessica walked back.

"Mike, why don't you shadow me for the first day?" she said. "I think it will help you gain some insight into the clinical workflow and the kinds of patients you'll be seeing."

The first patient was a woman with ongoing digestive problems.

"I've basically exhausted the workup for diarrhea," Jessica confided. "Can you think of anything?"

I asked the patient if there was anyone in her family who suffered from digestive problems?

"My sister was diagnosed with lactose intolerance," the patient said. "But I didn't think I could have that, because she was just a baby when they found that out."

I explained that lactose deficiency could manifest at different ages, even among siblings.

"Oh, yeah," Jessica said. "I should have thought of that..."

The next patient appeared distraught. Still, Jessica approached her, upbeat.

"Today you get two doctors for the price of one," Jessica said, cheerfully.

The patient complained of pain in her hand.

"I'm right handed," she said, "but now I'm having so much aching in the hand that I'm not able to use it, and I'm using my left hand more. I went to the emergency room, but they didn't do anything."

"Did they do an X-ray?" Jessica asked.

"Yes," the patient responded. "They said it was normal."

Jessica examined the patient's hand, then turned to me.

"What do you think?" she asked.

Removing a pen light from my white coat, I shined it against the skin of the patient's hand.

"It trans-illuminates," I said. "It's likely a ganglion cyst."

"What do you think we should do for it?" Jessica asked.

"I think the patient needs an additional imaging study," I said, "then evaluation by a hand specialist for possible surgery."

"I agree with you," Jessica asserted.

The patient became tearful, and Jessica moved close, then took her hand and stroked it.

"Don't worry," Jessica said, soothingly. "It will be all right …."

Near the end of the day, I followed Jessica to the end of the hall. At the door of the examination room, she looked at the name on the chart, then pulled me aside.

"The patient inside is mentally challenged, and has something of a crush on me," she confided. "So, don't be offended if maybe he doesn't like you coming into the room with me."

Indeed, when the man inside saw Jessica, his eyes instantly brightened, then darkened when he saw me trailing behind.

Jessica asked the patient questions, then reviewed the chart. The patient sat and watched Jessica.

"Do you have a sister?" he asked.

Jessica ignored the question and discussed adjusting his medications.

"I don't need medicine," he responded. "What I need is a girl like you…"

Leaving the room Jessica was pensive.

"Sometimes, I wonder what I'm going to do with him?" she said.

I smiled: Jessica was beautiful, so that I couldn't imagine anyone not attracted.

"I appreciated his honesty," I responded.

Returning to her office, Jessica threw her stethoscope over her shoulder, then bounced into her chair.

"Well, I don't think you need to shadow me anymore," she announced. "I appreciate your attitude of service, your skill and philosophy towards patient care. It's always been my position that you'll be an asset to the group…"

CHAPTER FOUR

Leaving the Health Center I joined my fiancée, April, at her grandmother's.

"How was your first day?" April asked.

I told her about the staff meeting, then the conversation with Lang. April frowned.

"I don't get a good feeling about that place," April said. "That first day when you were bringing your paperwork for credentialing, that woman was rude to you... Just the dismissive, unhelpful manner you were treated – sending you to a 7-Eleven miles away to make another copy for them, when there were all those copy machines right there. And this is the way they treat their doctors? On the first day when they should be trying to make a good impression? Do you really want to work here? I just think there's something wrong."

It was just one member of the staff, I said. It didn't represent the entire organization. Probably just a person having a bad day.

April wasn't convinced.

"I got bad vibes," she said. "I'll never forget this one doctor I saw there when you brought back your paperwork... You had to go to a different room to complete it, and I was sitting there in the office, and this other new hire came on. He was a doctor like you, and he was coming in for his first day on the job. And you should've seen him – He walked in there, and he was so hunched over. He was holding his hat and his briefcase, and he was holding it so close to his chest – He was like a little rabbit or something. And I was like, 'He knows it, too. He knows he's among predators - And he's a prey.

"And maybe that's why they hired him? Maybe that's why they hired you? You can give off a feeling like, 'I'll go along with whatever you can hand out.' But I don't think people realize that there is a wall that, if you hit it, there's no breaking it. No stepping over it. You won't bend."

She took a deep breath.

"I was talking with grandma about it today," she continued. "For years she worked as a social worker in a clinic not far from where FQHC set up. You know what grandma said about them?... 'That place swallowed up our clinic. We didn't like them. They were predatorial.'"

I looked over at April's grandmother; at 96-years old she was frail and infirmed, and I wasn't inclined to take such thoughts seriously. But April was insistent.

"I think grandma knows what she's talking about," she said. "It's not too late to find someplace else."

I thought about Lang's comment of 'winding up on an Indian Reservation', and how I'd held back from saying I'd been offered a job serving native peoples on such a Reservation, and it was only because of April's grandmother that we'd come here.

"Call them at the Reservation," April urged, "and say that you changed your mind, and want to work there after all."

I shook my head.

No, I'd made my decision. I was a well-seasoned physician, unafraid of hard work or long hours. I had no doubts about my medical competence and professional ability, and especially not my ability to care. Throughout my career, I'd never shrank from taking on the most difficult challenges. Straight out of Residency, I followed a girlfriend to Tennessee and took over for a doctor with the worst mortality rate in the hospital, and left there with a reputation for saving lives. In my previous position as a Medical Director with the Tennessee Health Department, I'd accepted a position at a community medical center that was rated worst in the State, and transformed it into a recognized model of excellence. There was nowhere I couldn't succeed, thrive and be appreciated. It was just a small matter of time.

CHAPTER FIVE

The following day a patient complained of persistent cough despite repeated visits to the Health Center.

"I've been coming here for the last six months," he said. "Every time I come here, I see a different doctor, and he just gives me another antibiotic and sends me home – and I'm not getting better…"

"What did you do for him?" April asked that evening.

When I'd listened over his lungs, I heard a 'whistling' at the left base. I ordered a chest X-ray and it showed a tumor on that side.

"What will happen to him now?"

I ordered a CT guided biopsy. If it's malignant, with luck the tumor will be confined to the lung and completely removed by surgery.

April was quiet, then turned and kissed me.

"I'm proud of you, Michael," she said. "You might have saved a life   today…"

CHAPTER SIX

Visiting April's grandmother Friday evening, the snow was falling heavy, so that after dinner, it wasn't safe to leave. The grandmother was attended to by a caretaker named Lisa, who kindly arranged the spare bedroom for April and me to sleep in.

"It's hard to make a lot of space," Lisa said, "because Marietta [the grandmother] keeps everything. She has gas bills from 1973. Me, I pay the bill, and after 3 months, I throw it away. She has things that are a hundred years old… You think I'm kidding?… Look over here. In this box there's a passport from when Marietta came over here from Czechoslovakia in the 1930's. Here's something that Marietta wrote about her mother. Look at this."

I want to write about my mother but I am finding it much more difficult. I am not sure why. Maybe because I feel guilty. I think I gave her a very hard time, especially during my adolescence. At that time I was an intellectual snob and I looked down on anyone who was not interested in my intellectual topics…

Gazing up from the note, I looked in the direction of the grandmother, and tried to imagine her as this precocious little child.

My mother was a simple woman who had an 8th grade education as was the usual custom for girls at that time. She was loving and totally devoted to my father.

My mother's name was Ida Schlosser. She was born in 1875 in Prague. I do not know much about my mother's early years. I think she was quite overwhelmed by the boisterous and somewhat undisciplined younger brothers. I think she was pretty as a young girl and she proudly told me that she had long blond hair and beautiful regular teeth.

Her life was dominated by the prevailing tradition that a girl was expected to learn domestic arts and to wait for a suitable man to get married to. A 'suitable or acceptable' man was understood to be Jewish, already well established and preferably wealthy.

When she was sixteen, my Uncle Rudolph, was falling behind in his studies and my grandmother asked the director of the Jewish orphanage to recommend a tutor. Dr. Stern recommended a young law student, Fritz Eidlitz.

Fritz came and all the children fell in love with him. For my mother it was love at first sight. She adored him from the minute she met him and she knew that he was the man for her...

Sifting through more contents from the box, I found a letter that appeared to have been written on an old style typewriter labeled, From dad, Prague, October, 1941:

We are happy about all your efforts for us. We got your telegram about the visa to Cuba, but the Cuba delegation is in Berlin, Germany and we would have to go there to get the visa. We have to finish our preparations in Prague to get the passports and that will take still several weeks. The Jewish community will pay for our passage on the ship. So we do not have to worry about that expense. The second difficulty is to get the permission to leave and that is more difficult to get. We will do what we can to get permission and we will let you know by telegram. We thank you for the many efforts and we are happy to see you soon...

Then, a curious handwritten note.

Can you go home again? 1933 Hitler elected. 1938 Austria. Sept. 1938 Munich – Chamberlain – 'Peace in our time'- Sudetenland. Jan. 18, 1939 we left. March 15, 1939 Hitler in Prague...

Finally, tucked away in a corner was a stack of papers that carried a more ominous subheading:

Letter from Gerta Schlosser, wife of my cousin Gerd Schlosser, dated October 10, 1945, answering my urgent requests for a report of what happened to all my relatives in the Holocaust. Gerta was the only one who survived...

CHAPTER SEVEN

April came into the room.

"Who's Gerta?" I asked.

"Gerta was married to Gerd," she responded, "my grandmother's favorite cousin growing up."

Dear Marietta,

I have received today your second letter and I am ashamed to have left you so long without an answer. The reason is that I was always a little afraid of writing to you of the dreadful things I have to tell you.

In January 1942, Gerd and I went to Terezin [a ghetto established by the Nazis for Jews in Czechoslovakia]. It was rather bad there in the beginning, we were in barracks, men and women separately, when Gerd wanted to see me, he had to carry trunks when there was a new transport, or to push a coal wagon and unload the coal, then he would get an hour to be together with me, or I had to go peeling potatoes in his barrack (stealing potatoes as well, for we got little food) or to go and scrub floors.

It was not easy to get there anyhow, you needed 'protection' and a lot of energy. Later on Gerd got a 'Durchlasschein', i.e., a permit, because he was working as an electrician, so he could see me more often. It was only after the evacuation of the Aryans from the town that we could circulate freely.

I think that your parents [Fritz and Ida Schlosser] arrived in April 1942. Uncle Fritz didn't feel too well because of his prostate, but was well looked after by Era Klapp (who didn't survive, but his old parents are alive).

Your parents were rather 'lucky' for they lived in the same house, side by side, in one room the women, in the other the men, so that they were together all day. Gerd was very often with them. Later, when we were allowed to walk in the town, we went there together. Uncle Fritz was always the same, joking and full of optimism.

In spring 1942 came also Victor and Edie [the grandmother's Uncle and Aunt] to Terezin. Gerd tried everything to keep them there, but it was not possible. The whole transport, with a few exceptions, went to Poland. We were very upset for it was only vanity on the part of one of the leaders that prevented their staying. Karl [another leader], who held a good position there, had tried his best. By the way, Karl with his wife returned and are living in Prague. Karl was very ill, an ulcer, his wife was ill too, with the lungs. Gerd was never one day ill, yet you see, it was always the most improbable that happened.

Victor and Edie were very courageous. I admired Edie. They were smiling and optimistic.

A few months later came Herta [Victor and Edie's daughter] with her husband, Emil, and son, Hansi. You can imagine how disappointed Herta was when she found that her parents were not there.

The boy got scarlet fever and so Herta and Emil stayed there, else they would have gone immediately to Poland. Hansi was very proud that he 'protected' the family.

I grew very fond of Herta, for I saw that she was genuinely good; in Terezin, most people had altered or showed their real self - but Herta remained as she was...

In spring 1943, there were many transports leaving Terezin, and your parents had to go, too - I am not sure about the date. Gerd tried to plead Uncle Fritz's illness, but nothing could be done.

Herta and I packed for them, for Uncle Fritz was still discussing with the leaders and Aunt Ida was so flustered that she could not do anything. Uncle Fritz didn't lose his humor, though, and when Aunt Ida saw it, she became more courageous.

They said this was a very good transport that went to Silesia [in Germany], and we were glad it wasn't Poland. But they were lies. Most of us were silly enough to believe those things. Only Gerd never believed them. But, then, he didn't believe the bad things either - and they were true...

I looked in the direction of the other room where we'd left April's grandmother, thinking I'd just read the pronouncement of the demise of her parents, and pondering the anguish and horror and loss she must have experienced on reading that!...

Friedel [Gerd's nephew] was in Lipa since 1940, at a farm where Jewish boys had to work. It was the greatest blow for the parents to be without Friedel.

Then, in summer 1943, Friedel came to Terezin to the joy of all of us. He had become a very handsome, broad-shouldered, tall boy - very intelligent. Really, a fine boy.

So our family was together for a short time, but we knew it wouldn't be for long. In September 1943, there was a transport again, and Gerd's parents had to go. Twice already, we had succeeded to get them out of previous transports; but this time, nothing was to be done. So Friedel went with them voluntarily...

Just then, April gasped.

"The grandson went with his grandparents," she said. "To the death   camps..."

CHAPTER EIGHT

Meanwhile, conditions in Terezin had improved considerably. 'It is too good to last,' Gerd said.

In September 1944, they came with a new gigantic swindle. They said they needed working transports of young men, a new camp was supposed to be founded in Saxonia. So when Gerd had to go I didn't mind too much, for we thought the end was near and I believed Gerd would be better off in Germany when the end came than in Terezin where they could do to us what they liked.

But Gerd must have had a premonition, he was terribly sad when he left me, worrying about me. All young women were very unhappy, so the Germans were so 'kind' to allow us 'to join our husbands.'

I didn't go voluntarily, I knew that Gerd would be against it, but when I got the convocation I was quite enthusiastic and left though I could have stayed, as I was teaching the wife of the Jewish Alderman [mayor overseeing the ghetto].

He was the 3rd Alderman. While the others were fine men whom the Germans made disappear, he was a swine and he is now in prison.

We went to Saxonia alright, but we went through it, traveled all day and all night, penned together like cattle and arrived in Auschwitz.

I must again ask your forgiveness. I had stopped because I was tired and lacked the courage to continue.

Well, in Auschwitz they told us to leave our luggage in the train and then came the famous 'selection' of which you have probably heard. There stood a medical officer and made signs with his thumb. Left meant life and right meant death, only we didn't know that at the time. Though I wanted to go to the right side, to follow a friend of mine, he sent me to the left.

All the children, and there were many and beautiful ones, with their young mothers, and the weak and the old people, were sent to the right side.

When we entered the gates and I saw endless rows of barracks closed on electric wires I didn't believe I would ever get out alive. Then, they led us to a bath where we had to undress, cut our hair everywhere, gave us some dirty rags and wooden slippers.

And now began a life that seems to me like a nightmare, no, worse, for my poor brain could never have invented such things.

But I was lucky. After a week already we were selected for work and sent to Freiberg in Saxonia. We worked there in a factory for 8 months. Hard work, little sleep and less food, only one dress, one pair of sneakers, one chemise [undergarment], no stockings. In February I got a pair. And yet it was paradise compared to Auschwitz.

The worst thing was that I didn't know anything of Gerd. But I was convinced that he would survive it. And this thought helped me to endure everything.

After all I heard later, he wasn't even given a chance to survive it, he must have been sent to the wrong side immediately. I can't yet understand it. There were many who after 8 months of a hell of a life were dying of hunger. In this case it was better to find an end at once, that is my only consolation, and yet - – but there is no use in speaking about that.

When the front was quite near the Germans packed us in coal wagons, with coal dust an inch thick, and for days and days we were on the road, never knowing where we were going, 60 to 100 people in one wagon, starving.

On the 13th day I escaped near Klatovy. The others still went for 3 days to Mauthausen concentration camp where we were to be gassed. I was hiding in a small village for 14 days.

Then the Americans came and I could go to Prague, sure Gerd would be already waiting for me. It was a wonderful thing to have a bath, to sleep in a clean bed, to eat as much as you like. I ate enormous quantities. But it wasn't the homecoming I had expected. Everyone you had known – and loved – gone. A strange town.

Now I have a flat, I am teaching as before, earning my living quite decently. I am even laughing and joking and most people think I am leading a content life.

Here you have the whole story. If you want to know more ask me, this time I will answer promptly. It was only the first letter that was so hard to write. You don't know how glad I was to get news

*from you and to know there are people out to whom you somehow
belong. Write to me soon about your life and your kids. I am so glad
you have them. If it is possible send me photos. Much love.
Yours, Gerta.*

Behind the letter was an official looking document that read as
follows:

Dear Friend,
    *Upon your request we have effected the necessary inquiry and
according to our card index of all inhabitants of the Terezin ghetto,
we have found the following data concerning the persons in question:*
    *Mr. Friedrich [Fritz] Eidlitz [the grandmother's father], last
residence Prague, was deported 2.7.1942 with transport AA1-651 to
Terezin, and 15.10.1942 with transport BV-1499 to Treblinka – did not
return.*
    *Mrs. Ida Eidlitz [the grandmother's mother], last residence
Prague, was deported 2.7.1942 with transport AA1-652 to Terezin, and
15.10.1942 with transport BV-1500 to Treblinka. She did not return.*
    *Mr. Oskar Scholosser [Friedel's grandfather and Gerd's father],
last residence Prague, was deported 27.7.1942 with transport AAu-502
to Terezin, and 6.9.1943 with transport DM-3161 to Auschwitz. Did
not return.*
    *Mrs. Marta Scholosser [Friedel's grandmother and Gerd's
mother], last residence Prague, was deported 27.7.1942 with transport
AAu-501 to Terezin, and 6.9.1943 with transport DM-3160 to
Auschwitz - did not return.*
    *Mr. Friedel Schlosser [young cousin to the grandmother], last
residence Prague, was deported 13.5.1943 with transport Db-28 to
Terezin, and 6.9.1943 with transport DM-3189 to Auschwitz - did not
return.*
    *Mr. Gerhard [Gerd] Schlosser, last residence Prague, was
deported 30.1.1942 with transport V-635 to Terezin, and 28.9.1944 with
transport EK-2497 to Auschwitz - did not return.*

"Each of them was taken away in a different transport car, and
probably went to the gas chamber alone," April said, "and met that
terrible death – of not being able to breath - without a family member
to comfort them."
    She shook her head and cried.
    "All of these people," she concluded, "that my grandmother
loved..."

CHAPTER NINE

"During the night my grandma tells me that she still sees the faces of her family," April said. "At times grandma says she looks at me, and is reminded of them. She says it's because I look a lot like the people in her family who she lost."

"I don't think grandma's ever come to terms with the way they met their end," she continued. "When my sister was in high school, she wanted to participate in a certain Holocaust program. It was called 'The Death March', and involved walking between the different concentration camps in Europe, and ended in Auschwitz.

"My parents didn't have the money to pay for it, so my sister went to my grandma, and asked for her support. Grandma had always encouraged us to learn about the world, and would, at times, help finance our travels.

"But, this time, grandma refused. She was adamant, and insisted that my sister not go on this trip, saying that the only thing she'd find there was death and graves..."

By morning most of the roads had been cleared, and April's mother, Doris, joined us at the grandmother's. April and I shared the contents of the box that we had discovered, especially the Holocaust letter. Doris read it, tearfully.

"This letter affected me, too," Doris said. "After my mother received it, she was so stricken by grief that she took to her bed, and wasn't able to care for me for almost a year. I was three years old then, and all I remember was the sound of her crying..."

Doris asked if I understood the significance of the grandmother's hand-written note about Sudetenland? I said I supposed it was her mother's way of recounting the critical events leading to World War II. She shook her head.

"It wasn't really about that, Mike," Doris said. "The Munich agreement was terrible for the world, but actually provided the way for my mom to get out of Europe.

"You see, her husband – my dad – had been born in Sudetenland. When Chamberlain signed the pact with Hitler that handed the Sudetenland over to the Nazis, it automatically put the Jews there at risk. That meant that they could apply for visas to the United Stated, and get out; the rest of the Jews in Czechoslovakia couldn't do that because they weren't considered at risk from Hitler – not until it was too late.

"No one else on my mother's side of the family had a connection to Sudetenland – only my mother because of her marriage to my father.

"There was actually a very narrow window for my mom and dad to get out – It was only a couple of months between the Munich agreement and the time when Hitler invaded Czechoslovakia.

"But my dad foresaw what was coming. He'd been a student in Germany for a time – and been thrown down a flight of stairs. So, when he got the chance to leave Europe, he took it in a hurry. That's how my mother became the only blood relative from her family to survive..."

CHAPTER TEN

While April and Doris attended Marietta in the other room, I continued sorting through the box, and found a copy of a letter dated 7-12-93, written to April.

I understand that you are thinking of spending a few days in Prague on you way home from Israel. I think that you will find Prague to be a beautiful city with both an ancient past and a vibrant present.

With your artist's eye you will appreciate the beautiful architecture of many of the century old buildings and you will love the hustle and bustle of the modern city with its tourists from all of Europe, especially teenagers and young people camping all over the city.

You will love to listen to the street singers who set up camp on the sidewalks with their guitars, sing old and new songs and ask for donation. You will love to walk along the big river called Vltava or Moldau as I and your grandpa Richard used to do every night.

You will go to the square in the old city and watch the famous clock with beats every hour and the 12 apostles appear and march around waving. The gruesome story of the clock tells that the inventor was blinded by the king so he would not be able to make another clock just like it.

You will go to the old Jewish cemetery where the grave stones are put one on top of the other because the graves are placed up to 10 layers deep in the limited space and you will visit the 500 year old synagogue.

You will see the statue of the famous Rabbi Loew, the legendary creator of the Golem, supposedly an ancestor of your grandfather Richard.

You will visit the 1000 year old castle of the Czech kings which dominates the city and you will go to the gathering place for painters and other artists who work there. However, wear a money belt under your clothes for your valuables! It is also a gathering place for pickpockets!

You will meet Gerta Schlosser who was married to my cousin Gerd and who is the only survivor of my family. She is about 85 and partially blind but she is very alert, speaks good English and will love to see you.

Have a wonderful time in my old playground!

Love   from   grandma...

CHAPTER ELEVEN

"Mike, if you're interested," Doris said, "I can put you in touch with more people who are Holocaust survivors."

I would be interested, I responded

"Alright, then I'll make some call," she said…

"My mom takes these things very hard," April confided. "She was born during the war. In that way you might say that she's a first generation survivor herself. How is she any less of a first generation holocaust survivor than her mom?

"Her mom didn't actually experience the Holocaust first hand. She wasn't in the camps. But she is a survivor in that she was a targeted group. But she got out before. And she suffered those losses. And she knew if she had made a different choice, she would have been in those camps. But she physically was safe and sound here in the states will the war was going on."

I thought about my reaction to first hearing about Holocaust; the dark cloud that seemed to settle over me when my mother told me that we were Jewish, just like those who perished in the gas chambers.

I shook my head.

First generation, second generation? I thought. How could it not affect you no matter how you're related?

"My mom often talks about being emotionally wounded as a child by her mom's trauma," April continued. "She could really use some healing from the circle of trauma that she got from her mom. Me, too. I was reading an article about third-generation survivors, which I am, and they were saying that on a broader trend, the way that the Holocaust affected the third generation is that they're finding they often have anxiety, and some kind of anxiety-related syndrome.

Panic attacks or generalized anxiety or something. They tend to have more issues with anxiety then the general population has. And I think, 'Yeah, I have that. I'm a worrier. I worry, worry, worry'; so I can see that in myself. I'm a typical third generation that way…"

Placing the letters back in the card-board box, I stumbled upon a final note – one titled, 'An important day in my life.'

It was January 26, 1939. I was in the cabin of the French ocean liner Isle de France, lying on my bed desperately sea-sick. It had been a very rough crossing on the stormy Atlantic. I had been sea-sick most of the 6 days since we had left the coast of France. I was traveling with my husband to the United States, leaving our old life behind and embarking on a new and exciting adventure.

It had been a difficult decision to leave my native Czechoslovakia. We had a happy and fulfilling life in Prague, the beautiful Capital of our country. I was a teacher and law student and my husband was establishing his medical practice as a pediatrician. We had a large and loving family consistent of parents, brothers and sisters and many aunts, uncles and cousins.

Leaving the country was an idea which was furthest from our minds. But the clouds of war and political upheaval were closing in on our peaceful democracy and many of our friends were preparing to leave.

Young and adventurous as we were, we decided to go away for a short while and return when the political situation improved. This was a very naïve and simplistic idea. We did not anticipate that we would never see our family again. That a devastating war was going to engulf Europe and that 50 years would pass before I would again set foot on the beautiful ancient city of Prague.

As I was lying in the cabin, sick, and feverish, I heard a noisy commotion outside, cries of, 'There she is,' and, 'Look how tall she is.'

The ship was shaking violently in the heavy surf and I had to make a great effort to get out of bed and climb upstairs on to the deck. I had seen many pictures of the Statue of Liberty but I was not prepared to see it close up silhouetted against the New York skyline. It was an awesome and exciting view.

We finally landed in a heavy winter storm and started our new life in a new land, with a new language and new friends, but I never forgot that first impression of the United States with the great Statue in New York harbor greeting us with outstretched arms of welcome…

CHAPTER TWELVE

In the examination room, an older patient was seated. He was seventy years old, the possessor of gray hair and pleasantly distinct, well-chiseled features. He resembled my grandfather's in his later years, though (unlike my grandfather, who suffered from Alzheimer's) the patient's mind was sharp. In turn, I thought he was lucky — as were his children and grandchildren — that he had all his faculties, and perhaps always would.

"I just need a refill on my pain medication," he said. "I use it for problems with my back."

He handed me an empty bottle. It was Hydrocodone – a narcotic agent. Considering his age and infirmities, I was happy to refill it. However, reviewing his chart, I noticed he hadn't had a urine drug screen.

"It's just a formality," I said. "Hydrocodone is a controlled substance, so everyone needs to be tested."

He went to the lab, then returned shortly after. I noted that he'd been treated with two different strengths of the medication — 5 and 7.5 mg.

"I don't want this one with seven milligrams," he responded. "I like the fives. I'm afraid of the higher Tylenol content in the first one."

I explained that both pills had the same Tylenol content.

"So, if you're worried about Tylenol," I said, "relatively speaking, you'd effectively be putting less Tylenol in your system for the same amount of Hydrocodone by taking the 7.5 mg tablets."

"No, I don't like the sevens," he insisted. "I want the fives."

Nodding, I wrote for the 5 mg dose, contenting myself with the thought that although it might not give him as much relief, at least it

24

was less likely to cause side effects.

Later, though, the results of the urine drug screen returned, indicating that my elderly patient had tested positive for cocaine.

"It can't be," I thought.

I phoned the lab.

"No mix-up, Doc," the lab technician said. "It's mandatory that all drug screens are directly observed. We repeated the study. It's been   confirmed."

I called the patient, but instead of him, a young-sounding fellow answered   the   phone.

"Max   isn't   here,"   he   said.   "I'll   give   him   the   message."
And   concluding   the   call,   he   snorted...

CHAPTER THIRTEEN

Entering the next examining room, I tried to collect myself.

"Hi Doc," the patient inside said. "How you been doing?"

I nodded and peered into his chart.

"Hey, is there something a matter, Doc?" he said. "You don't look so good."

"It seems that some of patients have been getting narcotic medications without following the usual pain-management protocols," I said, collecting myself. "All patients receiving narcotic pain medication need to sign a controlled substance agreement and provide a urine drug specimen for testing."

Then I noted that this patient was also being treated with narcotic pain medication, and had neither signed a pain agreement nor a urine drug screen.

"I can't make any urine for you now, Doc," he said. "Before I came here, I used the bathroom."

"I'll give you some water," I responded.

Still, he was hesitant.

"I was at a party a few days ago and one of my bodies offered me a joint," he admitted...

"So, what did you do?" Jessica asked upon describing the interaction.

I explained in this State, marijuana was still illegal and gave him a month to clear the cannabis from his system. When he returned for his next appointment, he'd have to undergo drug testing. If at that time he tested positive, his narcotics would be discontinued.

"You acted in good faith," Jessica said. "He hadn't signed a contract before this. You laid down the ground rules. Now, if he breaks them in the future, he knows that he's going to be cut off."

I nodded, though, still, the question lingered: What if he'd been lying about the cannabis use? What if he'd been selling or trading the narcotics for cannabis or other illegal substances, and those narcotics were winding up in the hands of young people and getting them addicted, and that's why he didn't want to do the urine drug screen?...

"He read you," April said softly. "He saw that you were troubled and feeling down about that last patient, and you're someone who cares about his patients, and he found a way to get in your good graces, and used it to his advantage."

"That's what drug-seekers do," she added. "That's how they play you..."

CHAPTER FOURTEEN

Laboring for a mineral company, April and I took turns diving to the bottom of the sea. With only a thin rope line to follow, I dove hundreds of feet, then spent hours raking the ocean bottom in pitch blackness. Resurfacing, I passed April descending, though in the darkness, we never met...

Awakening from the dream, I felt a growing sense of unease: Over and over I was encountering patients receiving narcotic medications from providers at the clinic without opioid agreements or urine drug screen; then, when I performed testing, they were repeatedly positive for illegal substances like heroin and cocaine...

"Mike, this unfortunately is what seems to frequently happen when the issue of chronic narcotic prescriptions come up," Jessica explained. "You could call the local DEA [Drug Enforcement Agency] agent, Jack Reynolds. He could tell you if the patient is legitimate or if he or she is a known drug abuser-misuser. He is also very helpful to talk to in confidence about these issues."

Calling Agent Reynolds, I began by describing the case of the elderly patient.

"Well, let me ask you this," he interrupted. "Did any of the patient's narcotic medication show up in the urine drug screen?"

"No," I said. "There was no hydrocodone present. Only cocaine."

he said. "The hydrocodone sells for a couple dollars a milligram."

"I still don't understand," I said. "During the visit, I noticed that the patient had been treated with two different strengths of the medication — 5 and 7.5 milligrams. When I recommended the higher dose, he said he didn't want it, insisting on the 'fives'. If he were paid by the milligram, why would he want the weaker strength?"

"I'm not surprised," Reynolds responded. "The 'fives' are worth more on the street. They're the blue tablets, and the addicts all recognize them. The 7.5 mg tablets may be more potent, but they don't have the recognition that the 'fives' do — yet. That's why most of the drug seekers ask for the fives."

I stayed silent. I would have never guessed.

"You got taken, Doctor," Reynolds concluded, smiling. "Is this your first time? … Well, don't worry. It won't be the last…"

CHAPTER FIFTEEN

Invited to a party, the hostess greeted April and me at the door.

"Are you a doctor?" she asked. "Because there's a psychiatrist here. Would you like to meet her? ... Let me introduce you."

The psychiatrist was a proper-looking woman who wore her hair in a tight bun. She spoke about her work, and I asked her thoughts on drug-seeking and addiction.

"Drug-seekers are common," she said. "In my line of work, I see plenty of them. When they ask for Valium and other benzodiazepines, I just tell them no, and that's usually the last I see of them."

"Yes, but I'd like to understand them better," I said. "I'm still struggling with a couple of recent patients. I mean, here I am their doctor — charged with caring for them — and yet, it seems they've tried to deliberately mislead me."

In response, the psychiatrist lifted her eyes to the ceiling and subtly shook her head.

"Excuse me," she said, and abruptly walked off.

Turning to April, I shrugged.

"I guess I'm being foolish," I said, "and I should know patients do things like this."

April hesitated.

"Do you remember the first time you were in love?" she said. "Did you ever act out of jealousy?... Being addicted to drugs is kind of like that. You do things even if they put your mortal soul in peril..."

CHAPTER SIXTEEN

Arriving at the Health Center Jessica pulled me aside. "Michael, I need your thoughts on something," she said. "We have a situation. There's this patient who was expelled from Health Center last year. He wasn't supposed to be able to come back here, but he was scheduled in error for an appointment with you today.

"I could remedy it in advance by calling and explaining to the patient that he needs to get his care elsewhere," she continued, "but we've now made this appointment and I'm not sure what our obligation is to the patient at this point — 30 days of coverage, second chance at obtaining his care with us? I don't know.

"I didn't take care of him before, but I know a little about him. He was a very verbally abusive, drug-seeking patient who repeatedly called on-call providers requesting refills of controlled substances, saying, 'Dr. Lang did it for me last week, so why can't you?' When he became confrontational and threatened staff, we expelled him.

"He may be a different person now, and perhaps he's learned from his experience, but I imagine that he will soon be seeking the drugs he has been using for years. I would suggest that he be given care again with the explicit warning that any behavior similar to behavior last year will result in a repeat expulsion.

"Michael,   do   you   feel   comfortable   seeing   him?"
"I'd   be   happy   to   see   the   patient,"   I   said...

CHAPTER SEVENTEEN

"So the deal is," Jessica instructed, "no narcotics, and he needs to agree to mandatory substance-abuse counseling. If you want, I'll go over this with him first. It's your call."

No, that's not necessary, I said. I understood.

"OK," she said. "Just remember, this really isn't clinic procedure. Once a patient has been expelled from the Health Center, they're typically out for good, and access here is not an option. The exception we're making for this patient is way outside the norm. We're going out on a limb to help him...."

Opening the door to the examining room, I found a middle-aged man sitting inside, doubled over, with deep furrows on his worn and weary face.

"I had three failed back surgeries," he said. "They wanted to do a fourth, but I told them I had enough.

"I went through physical therapy, injections, implantation devices, spinal cord stimulators - none of it was helpful. In between, my doctors gave me boat-loads of morphine, Vicodin, Percocet, valium, and I got hooked on the stuff.

"I only take Tylenol now, and just live with the pain. I don't want anything else. I just got out of drug rehab. They gave us lots of handouts. I brought some along in case you wanted to look at them."

He shared the stack of articles.

The problem of drug addiction is among the greatest challenges facing patient care. The reasons for it are varied. How do drugs impart an artificial sense of fulfillment? Addictive substances act on the pleasure system of the nervous system. After experiencing the artificial pleasure produced by drugs, nothing else compares.

For the addict, the drug has thoroughly ravaged the nervous system, so that the normal pleasures of life are thoroughly obscured and circumvented, usurped and supplanted by the addictive substance.

Without pleasure, there is little to live for, and we go through the day numb. Such is the life of the addict; the nervous system is so reconstituted and rearranged that there is no pleasure, except for those transient moments when he or she can get his hands on the drug. The addict is a shell of the person who he or she had once been; living for only one thing only — the drug — because it alone can   provide   pleasure.

Addicts lie to their doctors, deceive loved ones to attain money to pay drug dealers, and when they can't get their way by manipulating the ones who care about them, they resort to other means for procuring the funds necessary to support their habit.

I   handed   him   back   the   article.

"What   made   you   quit?"   I   asked.

"Got arrested," he responded. "After I got out of jail, my life took such a downward turn that I didn't have the energy to go back to   the   way   I   was   living   before.

"You never lose the craving, though," he continued. "Men will steal,   and   women   will   prostitute   themselves."

Then, his eyes met mine for the first time.

"You think we're bad," he said, "but ask yourself, Where is all this stuff coming from?... It's coming from doctors, that's who. For every 250 addicts out there hooked on the stuff, there's one doctor supplying   it."

He   lowered   his   eyes   and   reflected.

"If I had one wish," he concluded, "it would be to have my innocence   back   again..."

CHAPTER EIGHTEEN

Days later Jessica approached me, excited. "Michael, did you hear about your patient?" she asked. "The one who was expelled and then given an appointment with you?... He was found dead in his jail cell yesterday."

What was he doing in jail? I asked.

"He was sent there by the hospital," she said.

'Sent there by the hospital'?! I repeated. How could that be?

Jessica poured through the printout of the hospital summary.

"It says he was admitted for intractable back pain," she said. "According to the ER note he had an exacerbation of his condition when he sneezed while watching TV at home. He was just sitting on the couch at the time. An X-ray showed he broke one of the screws in his spinal fusion. Before he went to the hospital, he was trying to deal with it himself — just taking Tylenol. He hadn't eaten or drank anything for days."

Then, Jessica stopped.

"Wow!" she said. "They were giving him really high doses of morphine over there."

But why did they send him to the jail?

"It says he became combative," Jessica said. "Something about pulling out his IV and then swinging it over his head. They write he was discharged to jail as a matter of 'staff safety'."

I reviewed the lab tests performed in the hospital.

"He was in acute kidney failure," I said. "Probably because of dehydration from not eating or drinking for so long. Between that and the drugs, he was probably delirious."

I looked at the nursing notes.

"His vital signs were unstable," I said. "According to this, just before he was discharged, his heart rate was in the 130s. The kidney failure put him at high risk for cardiac arrest. With no one in the jail to monitor his vitals and kidney function, he probably suffered a fatal arrhythmia."

"Michael, notify the hospital," Jessica said. "We can't have our patients mistreated this way..."

CHAPTER NINETEEN

"So the patient became addicted through medical mismanagement of physical pain," April said after confiding to her about the case, "and was then 'discharged' - as in expelled - from the clinic due to addiction-related behaviors? And also sent from hospital to jail while critically ill? Unbelievable..."

After notifying the hospital, I was invited for a meeting of the Quality Management Committee where I was told the case would be presented. Entering the conference room, members of the hospital's medical staff sat around a large oval table - none introduced themselves.

"All right, Doctor," the hospital administrator began in an exasperated tone. "Why don't you just go ahead and tell us what you came here for?"

I looked about, confused.

"I haven't prepared anything to say," I said. "I was invited to attend this meeting with the understanding that the case would be reviewed."

The administrator looked to those around the table, and exchanged wry smiles.

"All right, then I'll start," he said. "First off, this case and all cases that come to this committee are handled internally in the hospital. Your health center won't be privy to any official response and there won't be any punitive actions taken against the hospital staff involved."

"The case you presented was reviewed," he continued. "The patient was in renal failure, but his potassium level was normal. Therefore, we conclude that actions taken were appropriate."

I've discussed this case was with a number of specialists, I responded. All of them had agreed the mortality rate for a patient in his condition was high, and predisposed him to cardiac arrest, which he likely died of in the jail cell.

An awkward silence followed, broken by the charge nurse.

"All I can say," she asserted, "is in my experience, I had never seen a patient that violent. He was the most violent human being I had ever seen."

"Whatever the patient's conduct," I replied, "where his life was in jeopardy, it was the hospital's obligation to continue treatment. You don't just discharge a critically ill patient - especially not to jail. Per the specialists I talked with, what happened here constitutes nothing less than medical malpractice. If you won't take action, you'll leave me no choice but to report this case to the Medical Board."

The eyes of those around the table hardened.

"Doctor, if you'll excuse us, we'll reconsider the situation," the administrator said. "Please wait outside."

For several minutes I sat alone before being called back in.

"Doctor, we'll review this case again," the administrator said. "But we'll be reviewing your cases, too, and we'll be letting you know if we have questions and concerns about the care you provide..."

CHAPTER TWENTY

At a dinner party I'd been talking about the difficulties of pain management at the Health Center when a woman approached me.

"Excuse me, I overheard what you were saying to that other woman," she said. "I take care of my father. He's disabled, and lives with me and my family. He takes a lot of pain medication, and I think he's addicted. The funny thing is, whenever his friends come over, he can be talking with them for hours and never asks for his medication. But as soon as they leave, he's crying about being in so much pain and hollering for his pain pills."

"Pain and depression can co-exist," I said, "so there's good evidence to suggest that much of the pain experienced by some patients is 'psychic' pain. To some extent, this might be the case for your father."

"Well, if that's the case, then why is his doctor just giving him more pain medicine?" she asked.

"I think it's because, in general, if a patient repeatedly comes to his doctor saying he's in pain and requesting stronger pain medication, then most doctors are going to advance treatment, and ultimately resort to narcotic agents," I said. "The most concerning side effect of those agents is addiction, because once a patient starts down that road, it can be very difficult to get off of."

The woman nodded and moved off. April had been standing next to me.

"I liked watching you the way you interact with people," she said. "The way you come into a room, and you smile and talk to everyone. You have this amazing gift for caring, and I just love that about you.

"Wherever you go, you speak to people from your heart. There's no beating around the bush with you, no holding back. You always strike right to the core of any issue. I love that about you, and I wonder if — as I'm around you — that won't rub off, and I'll speak my   mind   like   you   do..."

CHAPTER TWENTY-ONE

Arriving at the Health Center, Jessica approached me.

"Joe Harney called from the hospital today," she said. "He asked me to call you off. He said there could be no good to come out of a conflict and escalating divisions between the Health Center and the hospital. Already, they're holding up your credentialing there, so you don't have access to their electronic medical records."

"I know that it was me who told you to notify them," she concluded, "but now I'm asking you to pull back."

Who is Joe Harney? I asked.

"He's the Chief of Staff for the hospital," she responded. "Before he moved into that position, he was the Clinical Director here. He still sits on the Health Center's Board of Directors."

Why hadn't I heard of him? I asked.

Dr. Lang, who'd been sitting at his desk nearby, got up and sighed.

"Mike, you didn't want to hear of Joe Harney," he said. "Believe me, you didn't. You didn't want to hear of him, or hear from him."

He walked to the other side of the room, and then stopped at the doorway.

"The way you're going, though, you probably will," he concluded.

Lang left the room; Jessica sat frozen, like a prey animal that had just been alerted to the presence of a predator.

"Things were done a lot different when Harney was here," Jessica said. "Even I was handing out certain pain pills like water. We all did."

"When Harney left, I took over a lot of his patients," she continued. "There was this one. He was paraplegic. He'd been getting Percocet for years for decubitus ulcers. I performed a urine drug screen. There was no Percocet there. He'd been getting 120 pills a month. You figure, $10 a pill, and nothing that he had to put up front because the pills were paid for by insurance. Well, that's a pretty good return on your investment. For that matter, it was all profit."

She paused.

"We've made some changes since," she said. "But a lot of people still remember those days. I think Brad thinks about them. I can't say that I ever felt pressured to practice medicine a certain way, but other people did, and Brad was one of them. I think he felt forced into making a lot of hard choices. He had loans to pay and a family to support."

"'Loans to pay'?" I repeated. "'A family to support'? That justifies potentially getting patients addicted to narcotics, or putting them in the hands of people who would divert them? Jessica, there's a high   school   two   blocks   away   from   here."

"Mike, I appreciate your idealism," she said. "I've said that from the start. And I'm not asking you stand by and hand out controlled substances to patients who you think are diverting or abusing them. I support   you   in   what   you're   doing.

"I'm just trying to tell you that a lot has happened here. Brad saw   it.   It   wasn't   easy   back   then..."

41

CHAPTER TWENTY-TWO

Taking a walk April turned and stared in the direction of the street.
stalker."

Looking in the direction of her gaze, I saw what appeared as two black triangles that rose just above the curb. A moment later, a kitten lifted and bobbed its head; except for white paws, it was predominantly black.

"She looks like she has socks on," April remarked. "I think that's what I'll call her... Socks."

April made a clicking sound with her tongue, and the kitten sprang up and came to her, making circles around us.

"She wants to come close to me, so I can pet her," she said. "But she's a little scared, because she doesn't know if she can trust me."

Then, April's expression changed.

"She's been in some fights," she said. "There's a long scar down her ear."

Indeed, it appeared as though the kitten's ear had been sliced in two.

"Who knows what attacked her," she said.

I nodded. It seemed difficult to imagine, seeing how small she was — like a gentle ball of fur.

April looked overhead at the darkening sky.

"You know there's a storm's coming," she said. "There might be tornadoes, too. I heard over the radio that they were telling everyone who has outdoor pets to bring them inside. I don't know how she's going to make it through all that. You think we could help this kitten through the storm? I know we weren't really planning on having a cat, but maybe we can help this little thing through the storm that's coming."

April knelt and held out her hands, but the kitten kept her distance.

"It's probably because she doesn't know me very well," she said. "And I don't know her very well, and don't know if she's going to bite me or something."

April rose, looking pensive.

"I think I'm ready to go home now," she announced.

But walking back, April made the clicking sound, and the kitten followed, zipping back and forth in front of us as we made our way.

At the house April opened the door; but the kitten remained outside on the stairs, looking in.

"She wants to come inside, but she's scared," she said. "And we don't have any cat food. I always heard that if you give them a bowl of milk, they would like that."

April put a bowl just inside the door and poured some milk. The kitten sniffed at the milk.

"She wants to go in there and get it, but she's still scared," she said. "I can tell she's really hungry and wants it."

Then, the kitten got down low, and slowly inched forward towards the doorway. She looked outside, and then she looked at the bowl of milk, and then outside again.

"She's thinking, 'I want that milk,'" April said.

Finally, the kitten crossed the threshold and licked the milk.

But when April closed the door, the kitten jumped.

"Did you see that?" she asked. "I'm going to open up the door again so that she can go back out if she doesn't want to be in."

But the kitten stayed.

"She doesn't want to go back outside," April said. "Because it's nice inside and there's the bowl of milk here."

She closed the door again. This time the kitten didn't stir.

April went to the couch, and the kitten followed. As April sat reading a magazine, the kitten curled beside her and fell into a deep, exhausted sleep. From the other side of the room, I stood watching.

"What are you thinking, Michael?"

"I'm thinking there's nothing better than love in your life," I said...

CHAPTER TWENTY-THREE

The following day I received a call from Joe Harney.

"I regard your comments about my medical staff as inappropriate," he said, angrily. "Look, this is a tough place to practice, and these are hard times because of the workload. And, OK, maybe the cases you cited weren't our best work, but they've been discussed with the hospital VP, and we're going to make changes. One thing you might consider: If members of our medical staff are lost because of your complaints, there will be no hospital for your patients.

"Now, I'll do my best to discourage 'tit for tat' retaliatory behavior," he said. "But my staff feels threatened, so I can't give any assurances. Already, they've picked up a case and brought it to my attention. It concerns one of your colleagues at the Health Center. Last week, he treated a patient with an antibiotic when he presented there with chest pain — seems he thought the patient was suffering from pneumonia. Well, when the patient wound up in our emergency room over the weekend, we found he was having a heart attack, and by the time our cardiologists got to him, he required an emergency coronary artery bypass. I've already called your boss and given her the details. I told her I'd appreciate a full investigation, and we'd continue to be watching..."

Jessica confided that, indeed, she had spoken with Harney earlier; Lang was the doctor who'd attended the heart attack patient.

"Brad thought he saw an infiltrate on the patient's chest X-ray," she said. "To him it explained the patient's chest pain and supported a diagnosis of pneumonia. That's why he limited his treatment to antibiotics.

"In the official X-ray report, though, the patient's lungs were read as normal. The radiologist found no evidence of pneumonia. The spot Brad saw was just an artifact, and didn't represent an infectious process."

She rubbed her forehead.

"The medical staff at the hospital told the patient," she continued. "They said the doctor at the Health Center had misdiagnosed him, and it should have been obvious that he was having a heart attack, and instead of antibiotics, he should have been sent to the emergency room for immediate cardiac work-up; they claim it was our fault that the patient required emergency surgery, and it wouldn't have been necessary if we'd caught his heart attack early. I just got through talking with the patient's family. They came to my office to lodge a complaint."

She shook her head.

"I was expecting pushback from the hospital," she said, "but I hadn't anticipated this..."

CHAPTER TWENTY-FOUR

"Sounds like the amoral see the moral as 'inappropriate'," April remarked of my conversation with Harney. "Perhaps, this is a compliment in disguise."

She laughed.

"Are you going to report them to the Medical Board?" she asked.

No, I said. They say they're making changes. We'll see how things go and hope they get better.

I turned and looked out.

"What's the matter, Michael?" she asked.

I shrugged.

It just seemed like such a fallacy, I said. We walk around like we're so indestructible, like we'll live forever; and, yet, we're so fragile. I was seeing it with my patients all the time now. Life isn't forever. There are no guarantees. You could be here one day and gone the next.

I turned back.

"Why don't we get married?" I said.

"Are you sure that's a good idea?"

I shook my head.

"I'm not much sure of anything anymore," I responded.

"You'll have to do better than that," she answered.

I looked at her.

"I know I love you," I said...

CHAPTER TWENTY-FIVE

At the Health Center a patient requested the narcotic medication, Percocet, for pain; however, a review of the Prescription Drug Monitoring system indicated he'd been treated with Suboxone, a medication for problems of addiction, and it had been prescribed by not one but two different doctors.

"They gave it to me by mistake," the patient responded. "They said it would help with pain. Afterwards, both of them apologized."

I requested a medical release to review these doctors' records, but the patient refused.

"No, I won't sell these guys out," he insisted. "One of them is a family friend. The other is a good guy who's done me a lot of favors."

Without that information, I said, I can't responsibly prescribe you a controlled substances.

"Well, then, can you give me some Valium?" he pleaded. "Just ten of them. Ten!..."

Later that day I received an email from the CEO saying he'd received a complaint from the patient and wanted an explanation for why I hadn't prescribed the controlled substances?

I'd been replying to his email when Jessica asked if she could read it? Backing away from my desk, she read my response.

"Would it be okay if I modify it?" she asked.

Sure, I replied.

She began furiously typing.

It's in the best interest of patients who need help with their substance abuse that we not put them at risk with or give them opportunities to divert narcotic medications...

"There," she declared. "Send that..."

The days passed and I didn't hear back from the CEO. Then, I saw that the patient was scheduled for an appointment with Lang.

Pulling Lang aside, I shared my concerns about the patient.

"Don't worry," Lang responded. "He won't get narcs from me..."

Not long after, though, a form from the patient's insurance company appeared on my desk, requesting an explanation for visits to a pain specialist.

Pain specialist? I thought. I didn't send him to a pain specialist. How did he get there?

I called the specialist.

"Yes, I'm aware that the patient's been treated with Suboxone," the specialist answered. "No, the patient didn't sign a medical release for me, either... Yes, I treated him with Percocet... I gave him Valium, too."

Who referred the patient to you? I asked.

"The referral came from a Dr. Bradley Lang," he responded. "I believe he works out of the same office you do..."

"What's the problem?" Lang told me. "The patient has Medicaid. Just because we won't prescribe narcotics to the patient, it has no relation to what the pain specialist does. As an outside office, they make their own determination about narcotics — they're not under our narcotics policy."

"But he's still technically my patient," I responded. "And now his insurance is asking me to justify the referral. And I still want to know if he has a problem of addiction."

"Mike, we're expected to do referrals," Lang quipped.

He   shook   his   head,   then   turned   his   back...

CHAPTER TWENTY-SIX

Traveling back from a perspective wedding location, April asked if we could stop at a pottery shop?

"They're having an evening event," she said. "I just want to see if it features the work of any of the artists I went to school with."

April's mother, Doris, was with us; as we walked about viewing the displays, by chance, we ran into the FQHC CEO, and I introduced him to April and her mother.

"Looking for wedding sites, huh?" he said. "I'd suggest the State Park."

April talked about her interest in the current healthcare debate, and desire to get politically involve. He listened with interest.

"We're having the State Senator speak at the Health Center," he said. "You should come…"

Doris had been mostly quiet, though appeared quite taken by the CEO.

"Who is he?" she asked after he left the shop. "He's the CEO for your clinic?!… I'm just surprised because he seems so young and energetic and full of idealism. I think he's a lot like you. It seems like the two of you are a good match…"

CHAPTER TWENTY-SEVEN

*SENATOR ANNOUNCES $1.2 MILLION GRANT FOR NEW
CONSTRUCTION — A senior member of the Senate Health,
Education, Labor, and Children and Families Committee, and
FQHC, Inc. Chief Executive Officer will announce today that the
center has been awarded a $1.2 million grant from the U.S.
Department of Health and Human Services. The funds will be used
to complete the expansion of FQHC's Abyssal Heights location. The
expansion will bring approximately 17 full-time construction jobs to
the state, as well as 13 full-time permanent health-care jobs to staff
the expanded location. FQHC estimates that the Abyssal Heights
expansion will enable them to treat approximately 2,000 more
uninsured and underinsured patients on top of the 10,000 they already
see annually...*

As the FQHC staff poured into the auditorium for the Senator's
reception, I attended a patient in my exam room.

"What do you think of national healthcare," he asked. "You are
in favor of such a plan?"

Well, it's complicated, I said. There's a lot to consider.

"Like what, Doc?" he said.

The cost of medicine is expensive, I said. Sometimes addressing
symptoms can involve expensive tests, and if patients don't have to
directly pay for those tests - and the taxpayer is the one left with the
bill - I don't know that the system can handle that.

"Well, is it better to just let guys like me suffer?" he said. "Just
because I've been laid off, and can't find work, and can't afford
insurance right now?"

Patients like you are forced to make a decision about your health, I said. I can tell you that it's better to get a test, but I have to leave it to you to find the resources to do it.

"But if a doctor recommends a test, and it doesn't get done, then the patient's life can be at stake, right?" he asked.

Not necessarily, I said. These days a lot of tests are ordered that aren't really necessary. In many cases, doctors are doing this to try to protect themselves against being sued.

"Well, do you think that's right, Doc?" he asked. "That people can't afford insurance just because docs are performing so many tests that they've driven up the cost of healthcare out of the reach of guys like me."

I didn't say I think it's right. I'm just telling you the way it is.

"Well, do you think it can be corrected?" he asked.

Yeah, it might. If there were oversight bodies composed of physicians saying, 'Based on these parameters, this test should or shouldn't be done,' then, yes, doctors would probably feel more comfortable not ordering as many tests. That way, if the physician were sued, he could say that he'd followed established guidelines.

"Well, that sounds like the right way to go to me, Doc," he responded.

Yeah, but there are other problems, too.

"Like what?" he asked.

Overprescribing. If everyone had insurance and they were going to their doctors because they didn't have to pay as much, there's a tendency for patients to be given too many pills.

"Is that the patient's fault?" he asked.

In general, when a patient comes to see his doctor, he expects he's going to receive treatment for his condition. That usually means a pill.

"Well, if a doctor feels like he's over prescribing," he responded, "can't he just tell the patient, 'No'?"

It puts stress on doctors to do that. There can be tremendous pressures out there for doctors to please their patients. Patient surveys go out, and a doctor's job in physician groups can be determined based on how well that that doctor is liked. It can even go as far as playing a role in determining how much reimbursement a hospital receives. All this can make it very difficult to tell a patient, 'No.' And if a patient comes looking and asking for the drug long enough, some doctors are going to give in, and feed a problem like an addiction, or worse.

"Well, maybe that's another reason why medicine needs to be nationalized," he said. "To make sure that all doctors are treating their patients responsibly and doing things right."

I nodded. Yeah, but that would take oversight and time.

"Then, shouldn't we start now, Doc?" he responded. "Before the problems you're talking about get any worse?"

I fell silent.

"Isn't it worth it, Doc?" he continued. "So that people aren't suffering, and we fix this system before it gets any more run down?"

Of course it is, I thought. Of course it's worth it...

As the patient left, I went to the auditorium in time for the Senator's concluding remarks.

"Federally qualified health centers provide critical medical, dental and behavioral health services to the thousands of underinsured people in our State," the Senator said. "In order for these centers to continue operating, they require critically important funding. I am pleased that FQHC, Inc. is receiving these federal funds to expand its locations so that they can increase their services and bring jobs to the area."

The CEO spoke next.

"During this economic downturn, FQHC has thousands of additional patients turning to us to provide them with needed primary care services," he said. "We hope to start construction within 90 days – so this award will help us address our patients' needs immediately. We are grateful to the Senator for his continued advocacy of meaningful health reform – as well as for the work of our organization..."

As the Senator and his entourage were leaving the auditorium, I held the door for them. Noting my white coat, the Senator stopped and shook my hand.

"It's a great honor," I said.

"The honor is all mine, Doctor," he said. "We appreciate what you're doing here."

I wanted to tell him about my conversation with the patient. But before I could utter another word, the CEO stepped in front of me, and led the Senator through a door and into the hallway...

CHAPTER TWENTY-EIGHT

With April's grandmother's condition deteriorating, the decision was made to involve hospice. I'd been concerned what that decision could mean, and asked the grandmother's longtime caretaker, Lisa, how things were going? Lisa responded that she'd been outraged at the conduct of the hospice nurse.

"She's holding a diaper, pulling on Marietta, and pushing me out of the way," Lisa said. "I said to her, 'You will not do that on my time.' She said, 'Yes, I will, and I'll do it again.' I said, 'I don't care if it takes six hours to change her bed. You do it easy and gently.'"

I shook my head.

"Maybe, she was in a hurry and wanted to leave," Lisa continued. "It was like she was saying, 'It's my job and that's it.'"

Visibly upset, April's mother interrupted.

"There is too much drama here," Doris said. "This whole conversation. There is too much drama."

"Michael is a doctor who wants to help," Lisa responded. "He's asking questions."

Doris was shaking.

"We need to support my mom's transition," Doris insisted. "We need to be giving her more medicines and keeping her comfortable. We do not need this conversation, and revenge against the hospice nurse…"

"'Revenge!'" Lisa repeated, insulted. "The nurse comes in here and… I can't do this."

Lisa left the room; I followed her outside.

"Mike, you don't know what's been going on here," she said. "Marietta's biological clock is all thrown off. I'm at my wits end. She

53

sleeps during the day, and then keeps me up all night, hollering and screaming and asking for coffee and food."

Terminal restlessness, I responded. There's treatment for that.

"No, Mike!" Lisa responded. "I don't want to drug her up. If I do that, she won't be awake for your wedding."

She shook her head.

"Michael, for the past months, that wedding is all she's been living for," she continued. "It's all she talks about. You might think that you know what's best, but I'm with that woman more than anyone. I bathe her, I clothe with, I sing to her, I wipe her after she's had a bowel movement. There's no one who spends more time with her than I do, and I listen to that woman. It's not just, 'Here's your tea. Now, let me put you in bed.' I've crossed all the boundaries that I'm not supposed to. And maybe I bud in where I'm not supposed to, but it's been three years, and I care about that woman and want to respect her wishes..."

CHAPTER TWENTY-NINE

The patient who'd been referred to a pain specialist returned to the Health Center.

"I'm feeling real shaky, Doc," he said. "I can't stop trembling."

The patient shook uncontrollably and looked as though he would fall out of the chair.

Have you ever had this problem before? I asked.

"No," he said. "Not even when I was drinking. I'd usually just wake up with a hangover. They just let me out of the hospital this morning. How long is this going to go on, Doc?"

I requested his hospital records, then discussed the case with Dr. Lang.

"According to the notes," I said, "his symptoms have required repeated emergency room visits and three admissions to the ward."

"And it hasn't been just the pain specialist whose been writing for his Valium," I continued. "The pharmacy record shows that you've been writing for them, too. I thought you were going to leave that to the specialist?"

"He came in a few weeks ago saying he was suicidal," Lang responded. "They were just fleeting thoughts. He had some dispute with his landlord. I gave him the Valium to calm him down."

Lang looked at me.

"Just write for some more Valium and send him home, Mike!" he insisted. "Tell you what, if you don't feel comfortable, sign the case over to me. I'll take full responsibility. No problem."

"His vitals are unstable," I said. "I've already given him two injections of Ativan, and his heart rate is still climbing. His pulse was 120 when he came here — now, it's 140. He needs to go back to the hospital. I've spoken with the psychiatrist there. He said that after

55

they get the patient medically stable, he likely needs to be admitted to a detox center..."

CHAPTER THIRTY

At an outdoor market I watched a woman carrying a small paper bag stroll to an outdoor café, and set the bag on the table where a man in a trench coat was sitting. The man pocketed the bag, got up from the table, and moved across town to a pier. There, he gave the paper bag to a second man. Then, in broad daylight, the first man pushed the second off the pier into the water. By the time I reached the pier's edge, the second man had already been carried off to sea.

Next, I found myself sitting in a darkened room; a number of dark-clothed figures were standing in front of me; I couldn't make out their faces, except for a central Godfather figure, who was sitting behind the desk across from me.

"Where did you see the woman with the bag?" the central figure asked.

I felt a strong sense of danger; it seemed that the only way I was going to get through this line of questioning – the only way I was going to stay alive – was to readjust my reality to his way of thinking.

"Tell you what, if you don't feel comfortable, sign the case over to me," he said. "I'll take full responsibility. No problem…"

I woke with a start.

"In the dream," I told April, "the Godfather figure spoke with Brad Lang's voice. He used the same words Lang did."

"Michael, it sounds like you have concerns about this doctor," she said. "First, one of his patients has a heart attack. Then, he writes for medications that wind up putting a patient in the hospital. You have to talk with your clinical director about it."

"It's difficult for me to judge," I said. "Maybe, there are times that patients with fleeting suicidal thoughts do well with a short course of Valium or other benzodiazepine. Maybe, Lang has significant experience with these sorts of cases..."

"Quit making excuses for him," she interrupted. "Would you have told a fellow physician to let a patient with symptoms like that walk out of the clinic? Michael, I know you like to think that all doctors are the same, but they're not. All of you pass the same boards and tests, but there are differences.

"If these had been your patients, you would be asking your colleagues questions. 'What do you think? What else could I have done?' Not, 'Give the patient some pills and let him leave.' Where is his Hippocratic Oath?"

I nodded.

"All right, I'll talk with Jessica," I said. "After the wedding..."

CHAPTER THIRTY-ONE

On the eve of the wedding, friends and family gathered for a dinner party; April and I sat between my uncle and confided feeling nervous about thought of marriage.

"Yeah," my uncle said. "Why ruin a good thing?"

April's father – a dignified man – sat alone. I approached him, and asked if we could talk.

"I think that the home that I was raised in was quite different from the home you made for your children," I said. "I don't know that I've ever seen a sustained relationship. I don't really know that I believe a relationship can last a lifetime. That kind of thing wasn't a part of my childhood experience. It wasn't what I grew up with."

He nodded.

"It was what you were taught," he said.

I bowed my head.

How do you un-teach that? I thought. How do you un-learn it?...

During the night, I sat in the shadows.

"What are you thinking, Michael?" April asked.

"I was hoping that this gathering of friends and family would help me," I said. "But, still, I have doubts."

"I have concerns about commitment, too," she said. "I'm an explorer. I never intended to settle down."

I shook my head.

"Maybe, we should cancel the ceremony," I said. "Tell everyone we decided to stay friends."

"Yeah," she responded, spiritedly. "'Enjoy the party!'..."

The following day, clouds obscured the light, and the caterers insisted that the ceremony be held indoors for fear of rain. But April objected, and the ceremony was moved outdoors again.

As we exchanged vows, April's eyes held me. If she truly had had doubts, I thought, it seemed she'd resolved them during the night.

Then, at the same moment that we completed our vows, the sun broke through the clouds, and even the rabbi appeared moved, smiling and raising his hands to the light, as though beholding some miracle.

"In the Jewish tradition, we conclude this ceremony with the shattering of a glass," the rabbi announced. "The origins of this ritual are not precisely known. Many scholars believe that it reminds us of the destruction of the Temple, so that even on the most joyous of occasions, we still remembered it."

The rabbi handed me the glass. Laying it on the ground, I knelt before it - a myriad of thoughts spinning in my head.

I don't know that I want a part of this tradition, I thought. Life is about creating, not destroying. Can I do this? Relationships, like glass, are fragile, and can be shattered in an instant. I'd seen enough of that. I saw what happened to Chrissie. He loved her. Could he have saved her?

Then, a thought – or spirit - entered my head, and I found the strength to rise.

That kind of destruction is within me, I acknowledged. It is for me to choose between creation and oblivion.

And then, with a force I knew not I had, a crashing sound rang out, and all cried in unison, "Mazel tov!..."

CHAPTER THIRTY-TWO

April's grandmother came for the wedding. I expected her to be out of it, but she was thoroughly awake for the ceremony, then for photos, and throughout the reception, actively conversing with family members who'd flown in from all over the country...

"You know what grandma told me," April said. "She said, 'You did the right thing. You waited for the right one...'"

I looked at Lisa, who forewent sedating Marietta with pills, and took it on her shoulders to pull Marietta through at the expenditure of time that she could have been comfortably resting and refueling what reserves of energy she had.

She was a stranger, I thought. She came into Marietta's life at the end. All of Marietta family perished – murdered at the hand of strangers. And here was Lisa, for whom the act of caring for another – a stranger – should be more than a job, but an act that involved giving   of   oneself...

CHAPTER THIRTY-THREE

For our honeymoon April and I traveled to a nearby beach town. In the evening while strolling the boardwalk, we passed a karaoke bar.

"Why don't you sing something?" April said.

We entered the bar. Most of those inside were young, and I couldn't imagine them interested in a song I'd pick. So, when my name was call, I was too nervous to look out at the crowd, and kept my eyes glued to the lyrics on the monitor. Finally, during an instrumental solo, I did look up; April was in the center of the dance floor, gliding along in a throng of young people.

"You didn't have to be afraid, Michael," she said. "I had your back..."

CHAPTER THIRTY-FOUR

Driving back from our honeymoon, I got a call from Brad Lang.

"Mike, the CEO is having a party at his vineyard," he said. "Most of the staff is going to be there. I think it's important that you show up."

Arriving at the vineyard I saw Jessica sitting at the CEO's table. She seemed quiet and restrained. Then, the CEO stood.

"I called you here to announce that yesterday was Dr. Sullivan's last day with us," he said. "She's taking a teaching position at the university, where she'll be training residents to enter firms like ours."

There was a gasp, followed by nods of approval. I stood numb.

"Our own Dr. Bradley Lang will be filling her position," the CEO continued. "He'll be our new clinical director."

Lang smiled as he accepted the polite applause.

I looked at Jessica still sitting at the CEO's table, and took out a sheet of paper, and began composing a letter.

As I look at you, I'm grieving, because I'll miss that blanket of protection that I've come to expect from you. You understand what is important to me, and even when it might not be your fight, you've been willing to stand behind me...

The CEO remained standing, as he described plans for expanding operations.

"We don't need a public option," he said. "National healthcare reform is already here. And its name is Abyssal Heights. The country doesn't want socialism. Abyssal Heights can provide medical care to anyone. How much more national could an option be? We accept all forms of insurance. For people who lack insurance, one day, we'll charge a sliding scale based on their income.

It's hard to come to terms with the thought of being without you, because even though I feel capable of meeting the challenges before me, it's not easy, and involves a kind of honesty and forthrightfulness and courage that means taking risks, and without your support, I feel scared...

"Our centers participate in the National Health Service Corps. This allows providers to pay off the expense of their education by working for us. And by lobbying for more money available to the NHSC, we'll increase this supply of physicians and expand the NHSC.

Naturally, there's only one answer — that's to cherish the gift that you've bestowed, and honor it by internalizing it, taking it into my heart, making it a part of me, and then letting it flow to others, so that they might be blessed I have been, and that core of giving that seems inherent in your nature — the purpose for which you were put in this world — might be truly honored, as I believe that you would want...

"All of this is happening in Abyssal Heights. There is no reason to believe this model can't scale up and provide care across America. FQHC is the national health care option that's already here, that already works, and, with it, we'll bring about the next generation of healthcare."

I'll miss you. I would have followed you anywhere. Because I believed in you...

Applause rang out at all the tables, as the staff cheered. I looked up at Jessica, and, for a moment, it seemed our eyes met.

But I decided I couldn't be sure, and crumpled up the letter...

CHAPTER THIRTY-FIVE

On my way out I passed Lang at the tiki bar.

"Congratulations," I said. "Obviously, the CEO thinks very highly of you. It looks like you have a good relationship with him."

Lang sneered.

"Alcoholics don't have relationships," he responded. "They have hostages."

I looked at him.

"Don't you know what the CEO was before he started the Health Center?" Lang responded. "He was a drunk, living on the streets. Everybody knew him. He was always going to the city council, complaining and talking about how something needed to be done for the homeless like him. When he said he was going to start a free clinic for he and the other street people, the council laughed, but thought he was harmless enough, so they gave him the clinic building.

"Then, he recruited Harney. Back then, Harney was mostly pulling late-night ER shifts at the hospital, doing what he did best — handing out Lortab, Vicodin and Oxycodone like candy. When the CEO hired him to be the first clinical director, Harney just brought all that to the Health Center with him.

"Business was booming, even if everyone in the waiting room looked like zombies. Then, they hit pay dirt .... They got the idea of making the clinic into a Federally Qualified Health Center. That's when the money really began rolling in.

"But instead of opening the doors to everyone — like they said they would — they only took patients with insurance. He talks about healthcare being a right; but, really, we take very few uninsured — there's no money in it."

He swallowed his drink.

"The CEO's very intelligent," Lang continued. "He's done well for himself. As well as the vineyard, he owns his own restaurant. He'll take you there and treat you — if you stick around long enough."

I'll be here for at least a year, I responded. I have that long to go on my NHSC obligation.

Lang smiled.

"Oh, yeah," he said. "The NHSC. I forgot. Yeah, they'll take care of you..."

CHAPTER THIRTY-SIX

Note to NHSC analyst:
Dear Ms. Cowley,
Just writing to say that things are going well in Abyssal Heights, and
that my fiancée and I married last week. April's grandmother has
benefited from April's presence here. We are looking forward to her
97th birthday this Tuesday, though she is in ill health. Recently, it was
elected to place her in hospice, though she still embraces every day,
as she certainly did during our wedding.
I continue to honor my participation in the National Health Services
Corp. In this time of national healthcare crisis it is important to me to
be doing my part for the country. Since my days of working on the
cancer vaccine at the NIH, I have valued work as a public servant,
and my affiliation with your organization is a source of pride.
 Sincerely,

"You didn't tell them about your concerns about what's going on at the Health Center," April said. "Don't you think they should know?"

I didn't think they'd be interested. They just want to know that I'm completing my obligated time.

"But you have a new boss," she said. "Someone who you don't have a good feeling about. Don't you think they should know that if something happens?"

Nothing was going to happen. Lang needed good, reliable doctors around him more than ever. I was rising in the ranks, and expected I'd only hold more sway in the future, and play a more commanding role at the Center.

April stared, then turned and shook her head...

CHAPTER THIRTY-SEVEN

At the Health Center an elderly patient presented with symptoms of stomach flu.

"I've had nausea, vomiting and diarrhea for a week," she said. "Now, I'm feeling dizzy."

The results of her blood work showed acute kidney failure.

"It's probably because your gastrointestinal losses have left you dangerously dehydrated," I said. "I need to send you to the emergency room now."

The following week the case manager came with an odd request for the patient.

"Doctor, I have a requisition here for you to sign," she said. "It's for this patient to receive continued dialysis."

"Dialysis?" I said. "What does the patient need that for?"

The case manager collected the notes from the hospital.

"According to the discharge summary," she said, "the ER didn't admit her when you sent her to the hospital. At home, her kidneys shut down, and when she was admitted to the hospital, her kidney function didn't recover. She's since required dialysis."

"Who was the doctor in charge at the hospital?" I asked.

"Dr. Smellin," the case manager responded...

I went to Dr. Lang.

"What's the big deal, Mike?" Lang said. "The patient has insurance and they'll pay it. It isn't like they're looking to investigate it or something. It's just a case where the patient wound up needing dialysis, that's all."

The dialysis will likely cost millions, I responded. And for something that should have never happened.

"Hindsight is 20/20," he retorted. "So they should have admitted the patient to the hospital the first time. So what? Are you going to threaten them again with going to the Medical Board? What's that going to do? You're only making relations with the hospital   difficult."

"No one cares about this," he continued, "Not even the patient. She doesn't know anything. No one's pointing a finger except you. And that's bad for business. Don't you know we rely on the hospital for patient referrals? Those referrals from the hospital are the life-blood of the Health Center. We need them to keep the flow of new patients. And your calls to the hospital are scaring them and threatening   to   dry   that   up."

"Brad, I'm concerned that Dr. Smellin is putting patients at risk,"   I   said.

"Of course he's putting patients at risk," Lang responded. "He's on call every other night and then puts in a full day at his clinic. If you were working that much, you wouldn't know what you were doing   either.

"Every time I see the guy at a hospital conference, he's asleep within five minutes of turning down the lights. But for now, he's the one volunteering for call at the hospital, and you just have to give him some   slack   because   he's   working   so   much."

"So quit stirring things up," he concluded. "You're just making things difficult for yourself and everyone else. I'm telling you to leave it   alone…"

CHAPTER THIRTY-EIGHT

Making my way from the parking structure to the Health Center, I saw an older man on a bicycle, and recognized him as the elderly patient who'd tested positive for cocaine on the urine drug screen.

"Hello, Doctor," he said, tauntingly. "I'm getting my care somewhere else now – where they don't make you do urine drug screens."

Riding on, he smiled.

"The less I see of you, the better I feel..."

Not long after, the office manager appeared at my cubicle.

"I got a call from the CEO," she said. "He says he wants to see you in his office — now..."

"I just had a visit with an irate patient of yours," the CEO said. "He said he'd been coming here for years getting pain medicine, and you asked him about using drugs."

"I'm sorry the patient was unhappy," I said. "Because of the narcotic use, I had to ask him to sign a Controlled Substance Agreement. Part of that discussion is informing the patient that a urine drug screen is requested, and if an illegal substance is found in that screening, the narcotic can and likely will be discontinued."

The CEO sat back.

"Doctor, you have to understand my position," he said. "I receive a visit from a patient, and it's hard for me to interpret if your explanation is legitimate. And, yes, narcotics are an issue with a few of our patients, but we have to be responsive and provide good customer service."

"I guess what I'm trying to say," he concluded, "is the Health Center has grave concerns about your care for our patients. Your approach to treatment differs greatly from that of the rest of our

medical   **staff..."**

CHAPTER THIRTY-NINE

Arriving home I learned that Marietta's condition had taken a sudden turn for the worse, and April had rushed to her side.

Spending the evening at her grandmother's, even at four in the morning, family was still coming in and out.

"I don't know where I'd be without her," a grandson, Samuel, said.

He held her hand tenderly and gently whispered, "We love you, grandma."

Marietta had taken to speaking in her native tongue.

"When grandma began speaking German," April said, "Lisa thought she was speaking gibberish. And this was difficult for us to hear, because up until then, her mind had been sharp. We thought, 'Oh, no.'

"And I don't know who figured it out – or how they figured it out – but, at some point, we realized that she was actually speaking in German, and she wasn't speaking gibberish."

"A little while later," April continued, "I was putting her to bed, and I stayed with her in her room, and we were talking so that she could go to sleep, and she looked around at me and told me, 'You look so much like them' – Her family that died in the Holocaust – 'But you wouldn't be able to talk to them because you don't know German, and they don't know English.'

"And then she goes, 'You know, they're over there in the corner.' And that's when I figured out why she was talking in German. It was because she was talking with her family members, and they were there in the room."

Samuel looked at me.

"Do you realize that she hasn't spoken that language since the War [World War II]?" he said. "Even though she was born and raised in Czechoslovakia, she was educated in multiple languages – among them, German. She worked with Sigmund Freud to translate his works from German into Czech. But she'd vowed never to speak German after learning the fate of her family in the Holocaust."

Samuel looked on, as though privy to a miracle.

"I think that she might be reconciling herself with the past," he said.

As the hours progressed, Marietta slipped into delirium.

Samuel turned to me.

"What's going on inside of her?" he asked.

Likely represents a confluence of worsening medical factors, I said. Infection, respiratory failure, heart failure, renal failure - all converging to produce this fluctuating state of consciousness.

"How will she die?"

The potassium will likely rise to levels incompatible with life, I said, so that the electrical impulses necessary for contractile activity of the heart won't be able to be achieved, and the heart will stop beating.

Marietta moaned.

"Why isn't she speaking?" he asked.

Internal changes, I surmised, likely affecting the brain centers responsible for speech and cognition.

"Does she know that we're here?"

It's possible. Delirium is defined as a state of fluctuating consciousness. Even though there are moments that she isn't with us, there are probably others when she's aware of our presence.

"I'm in a tunnel, and I can't get out," Marietta called out. "Take me home. Take me home."

Sam attempted to reassure her.

"You're at home, grandma," he said and pointed to photos of familiar family members that are everywhere in the room.

But Marietta continued to call out.

"I want to go home! Help me go home!"

'Can you go home again?' I thought, recalling Marietta's writings.

I administered the quick-acting sedative that the hospice service had provided.

"She willed herself to stay around this long because she wanted to be there for your wedding," Samuel said. "She wanted to see the two of you get married. For the past months, she'd been living for the wedding…"

At about seven I left for work. April stayed with her grandmother throughout the day and then through the evening.

Waking the next morning, I found April in the same place she was the night before. But whereas I was still shaking off the vestiges of sleep, it was as though there was a light emanating from her, and she appeared somehow refreshed, even though I knew she hadn't slept a wink.

"I just don't want her to feel alone," she said. "I want her to know that she's loved."

Marietta could never be alone, I thought. Had April been a thousand miles away, Marietta would have still been surrounded by the aura of her love, because April's heart would have found her anywhere.

"When all my female relatives left my grandma's bedroom last night," she said, "they were telling me, 'Leave, leave. Go, go. Go off to sleep.' But I was like, 'No, I can't leave.' So, I stayed here. And you were asleep in the living room. And Lisa I think was around in her bedroom. But I stayed in grandma's bedroom, and I was holding her hand. And she was already not totally there. She was still alive, but I think the morphine kind of sent her somewhere. But she was still conscious or something.

"So, I was here holding her hand, and from around midnight to about six or something, I was basically holding the hand of an unconscious person, that was still alive, but unconscious. But there was this really interesting energy transference I felt. I felt this very energetic joining from her hand.

"And it was interesting, because Lisa, before she went to sleep, said to me that singing might help. But out of some state of shock, I couldn't remember any song except, 'Row, Row, Row Your Boat' – which grandma actually liked. She used to sing that to me a lot. But that was the only thing I could think of, so I kept singing, 'Row, row, row your boat down the stream.'"

She broke into nervous laughter.

"All that chanting I trained in, and I was singing that," she said.

But that's what she was doing, I thought. Gently rowing down a stream, and life was 'but a dream.' It was the perfect song to sing to her.

"So, I was singing, and I was sitting holding her hand, and I was in this position where it was really easy for me to see that picture of her parents on the top of her dresser, and I really connected to that portrait – to them. I was talking to them. I was having these conversations with them in my mind. And I was sort of telling them,

'You were there when she came into this world, and I'm here when she's going out.' We had this bonding kind of thing."

"So, I think I did talk with them, even though they couldn't speak English, and I couldn't speak German," April concluded.

She stared in her grandmother's direction.

"Can you check on her?" April asked.

I felt Marietta's pulse. It was thread – notably different from the night before. Then, looking up, I saw that Marietta breathing pattern has abruptly changed, and recognized that she was going to pass soon.

"How do you know?" April asked.

I explained that her respirations had gone from regular to something called Cheyne-Stokes. I'd seen it before with my dying patients, and death usually followed quickly thereafter.

April rose.

"I got to go call my mom and everybody," she said.

I advised her not to.

"Why?" she asked.

Because they're going to get in their cars, and likely drive really fast, and potentially get in an accident, and they're not even going to get here in time anyway.

I move towards April and held her. Then, within three breaths, that flame which had burned so bright for so long was extinguished.

Lisa entered the house within a moment of Marietta's passage.

"What's happened?" she said, then shouted. "Hold on, Bubby, I have to get Doris down here first."

She ran frantic for the phone, then returned to the room, and knelt and wept over her lost friend's body.

Tears filled April's eyes, as she turned and held me.

"Thank you for being there for me and grandma," she said. "Thank you..."

Marietta Kohen, 97, of Coventry, died Saturday in the comfort of her home surrounded by her loving family. She was the beloved wife for 49 years of the late Richard Kohen, MD. Born in Pilsen, Czechoslovakia, she studied law at Charles University in Prague and was active there in the 'Blue-White' Zionist youth movement. She and her husband immigrated to the Boston, MA area in 1939 shortly before the Nazi occupation of Czechoslovakia. Her parents and entire extended family perished in the Holocaust. She worked in Abyssal Heights as a psychiatric social worker over many years with focus on healthy development of children. She had a passion for opera, theatre, tennis, swimming, travel and politics – she never missed a vote...

CHAPTER FORTY

Reporting to work, there was an email from the CEO.

Michael, in my usually quick read of the paper this morning, my eye was caught by the story/obituary of what sounded like a truly remarkable woman with an amazing life history. I realized this was your wife's grandmother, who I recall was the inspiration for your return here. I am very sorry for your family's loss, and happy that you had the opportunity to come and be with this amazing man during his final days. My deepest sympathies. I know how close she was in your wife's heart. May her memory always live with you both.

I shared it with April.
"Maybe it's a good sign," I said.
April was guarded.
"I wonder," she responded. "Do you think it was just by accident he came by this article about grandma in the paper? Or do you think it could be that they troll the newspapers for information about their doctors? — What they're doing, what they're saying? Then, use it to monitor it to decide who stays and who goes? Who they want to keep in their organization, and who they push out? Do you think that's possible?..."

CHAPTER FORTY-ONE

The scheduled morning patients at the Health Center had gone over, so I arrived late to the funeral. April was seated with family in the front of the temple. But I decided to take a seat further back, so not to disturb the ceremony. Lisa was seated nearby. Looking at her, I remembered the difficult conversations I'd had with her about Marietta leading up to the wedding. There were other caregivers at the funeral, too. Women who were not family, but had treated Marietta with utmost care...

"All of grandma's contemporary family members perished at the hands of strangers," April said. "Gassed in the concentration camps of Auschwitz and Treblinka. In that way you could say it's a source of hope that someone who could be described as a stranger came into grandma's life at the end and was such a source of support to her..."

CHAPTER FORTY-TWO

After the funeral service an older gentleman approached me.

"I hope your wife is alright with her grandmother's passing," he said. "I'm having some troubles... I lost my wife recently, and it shook my faith in God. I kept thinking, 'We're asked to pray that our names will be inscribed in the book of life. I prayed that my wife's would be, and yet she died. Why wasn't her name in the book of life? Why didn't God listen to my prayer?'"

I shook my head.

Can't know the design of God, I said.

"That's right," he responded. "Who knows if God didn't have a design in the Holocaust?"

I'm not willing to go that far, I responded. I think that was a choice that a lot of evil, misguided people made. But sickness, death – you treat people, you do the best you can, and if they die, you have to accept.

Doris had been standing nearby, and overheard the conversation.

"I still have questions about my mother's death," she said. "Mike, do you think that there could have been some divine influence that kept my mom alive till your wedding?"

I give most of the credit to her caregivers, I said. If they would have started her on the sedatives earlier, she wouldn't have made it.

Doris was quiet.

"I think mom willed herself to be at that wedding," she said. "She was that kind of person. After that, she didn't have as much reason to live. She knew the winter was coming, and she always hated the winters here. I think it was by choice that she died when she did."

"We really enjoyed your wedding," the man said. "What I was so struck by was that it was everything a wedding should be."

"You must really enjoy what you do," he continued. "There's always this spark about you."

I told him that I didn't know how much I enjoyed it. I believe in it. But sometimes it really keeps me up at night, especially now that I'm being confronted with questions of how I practice.

"It sounds like they want you to be a supplier," he said. "Are you planning on staying?"

Where I'd made a commitment to the NHSC, there was no doing otherwise. The question is, What do I do after that? Find someplace else to work, or stand up for myself and say, no, I want to work here?

"It's an old question," he said. "'When do you stand like an oak, and when do you float like a willow?'"

He was quiet.

"My wife died of cancer," he said. "She had ovarian cancer, and they'd only given her three months to live. She went through surgery after surgery, and chemotherapy over and over, and managed to survive for five years, and kept working that entire time, all the way up to the week she died.

"She was pretty lucid during those last hours. Before she died, I asked her, 'How did you do it all these years?' 'It's kind of like ping pong,' she said. 'Sometimes you're up, sometimes you're down. You go back and forth.'

"I told her, 'Well, I think now it's time for you to spread your wings and fly.' And that was the last thing I ever told her. She died later that night..."

CHAPTER FORTY-THREE

Leaving the temple with April, I suggested a walk in the park. We hiked along a stream until arriving at a waterfall. I stood in wonder, just as I had when I was a boy with my grandfather, watching as the falling water reached the bottom, and then cascaded down a natural staircase carved in the rock, 'til emptying into a meadow over-brimming with flowers.

"My grandfather would have loved this place," I said. "He loved the natural world. Used to quote poets on nature – 'I think I shall never see, a thing as lovely as a tree.' He so wanted to instill that in me. But I didn't appreciate it then. I wish he was here now."

I hesitated.

"When I was a kid," I continued, "and feeling down, he'd tell me as long as I followed my heart, I'd be OK and succeed in anything I genuinely wanted."

April was silent, and I wondered that talking about my grandfather at this time so close to her grandmother's death had been insensitive?

"Did your grandfather leave you anything?" she asked.

The question took me aback.

No, the fortune was left to my uncle, I said. He was the executor of the estate.

"Too bad," she responded. "Maybe, you could have paid off the NHSC and got out of your obligation to them, so you could leave the Health Center."

Is it that bad? I asked.

She was quiet.

"Michael, I know you want to help people," she said, "but for most of the patients who you're having difficulties with, it seems like you're trying to save them from themselves. And they don't want that kind of help.

"And you're working for an organization that doesn't respect what you're trying to do — because the patients are threatening to go somewhere else, and that's affecting their bottom line. They're about profits and pleasing their shareholders, Michael, and I don't think you're going to find a middle ground…"

CHAPTER FORTY-FOUR

"Patients are seen as customers," April continued, "and the customer is always right. That's why there's so much pressure on doctors to please this population, and very little consideration for doctors, especially when they're decisions displease the patients, creating a situation where bad medicine happens because it becomes more important to please the patient than perform responsible medicine.

"With as much concern as that the CEO wants you to apply to your complaining, drug-seeking patients who tell you you're 'unqualified', and walk out on you, he sure hasn't treated you with much concern..."

CHAPTER FORTY-FIVE

"Doctor, I'm calling because I hear you care about your patients, and I have a daughter in the hospital who is very sick," a concerned father told me. "I've been taking her to the Health Center and to the hospital for the past days, but nobody wants to do anything for her. She's in the hospital now. She has all this abdominal pain, but all they'll give her is Tylenol, and she's getting worse."

I asked for the daughter's name, then called the hospital and asked to be connected with her room.

"It's on my lower right side," she said. "I went to the hospital all weekend long, but they kept sending me away, saying it was nothing. Now, they have me sitting in this room and Dr. Smellin keeps saying I don't need anything."

I called the hospital again, and this time asked for Dr. Smellin.

"He isn't here," a nurse said. "I can take a message."

"Please ask him to call me," I said. "It sounds like the patient has appendicitis. Have imaging studies been ordered?..."

I called several more times. Although Dr. Smellin didn't return my calls, the nurse told me that he had received my message and ordered a CT.

"The CT showed the patient has a ruptured appendicitis," the nurse said. "They're in the room now prepping her for emergency surgery."

I went to Dr. Lang.

"The delay in care probably led to the appendix rupturing," I said. "Patients are dying under this man's care. I feel that to stand by makes us accessories to a crime. The appropriate authorities have to be notified."

"Wait a minute, Mike!" he said. "What if I told you I saw the patient the day before she went to the hospital? For your information, she had a D&C [dilation and curettage] after a miscarriage a couple of weeks ago. The other day, I gave her antibiotics because I thought she had a uterine infection. I didn't think she needed an imaging study, either."

"So, what are you going to do, Mike?" he concluded. "Report me now?..."

CHAPTER FORTY-SIX

The CEO collected the physicians together in the conference room.

"The last time I had you all in this room here, I talked about the importance of customer satisfaction," he began. "At FQHC, customer satisfaction is job one. It's our highest priority. I detailed why it was important and set expectations for you to follow. We have great examples of doctors who have proven records of customer satisfaction.

"Dr. Bradley Lang is a model of it. That's why I made him your clinical director. I know that our patients greatly appreciate his efforts, and so do you.

"But I have heard that some among you are not satisfying our customers. Some of you are not pleasing your patients, and that is unacceptable.

"You are not doing a good job if you are not pleasing your patients. Your job is to keep them happy. If you are not keeping our customers happy, then your style of practice is flawed.

"And customer satisfaction is not just an individual effort; it takes a team. Each of you should be supporting one another. This is especially true of your clinical director. There's something wrong when a member of our medical staff questions our clinical director. I regard it as insubordination, and it will not be tolerated.

"You should work together to improve customer satisfaction. If just one of you leaves a patient dissatisfied, the work of everyone is impacted. It's everyone's responsibility. If we don't have satisfied customers, we have nothing. There is nothing we can do to convince our patients we have provided quality health care if they are unsatisfied with our care.

"Customer satisfaction is a part of your evaluations. It's that way for a reason. It is the most important part of doing business for the firm. It is the right thing to do. You are not performing your job well if you are not making our customers happy.

"I am also going to encourage patients to give us more feedback on their customer satisfaction. Each of you in this organization needs to be willing to accept this feedback. If it is positive, keep doing what you're doing. If it is negative, make changes. If you do not improve, you will be held accountable.

"Complaints about poor customer satisfaction will not be taken lightly, and you should not be surprised to be disciplined. Remember, customer satisfaction is job No. 1 at Abyssal Heights."

"Nothing feels better than to have a patient smile and say thank you," he concluded. "Satisfying our customers is the way to change and improve healthcare..."

CHAPTER FORTY-SEVEN

At a gathering of the FQHC medical staff, pizza was delivered; but instead of sitting down for a meal, the physicians took turns sliding in the pizza, until we were all covered in it, looking as though soaked in blood and guts. Staring at the others, they were smiling and laughing, seemingly finding it exhilarating.

What are we doing? I thought. Is this supposed to be fun?

Children appeared, and the doctors in bathing suits now, slid the children down slides as thought at a waterpark; but instead of water, the slides were flowing with blood.

"This isn't right," I said.

But my colleagues just smiled and gave the appearance of having fun, while they and their families were covered in blood.

"No," I said. "This is wrong!..."

Awakening from the dream I sat up in bed.

"It's disgusting," April said. "The wholesale prescription of narcotics. The condoned malpractice at the hospital. What's happening at the Health Center is absurd."

"Mike, I'm ready for a change," she continued. "The Health Center is being hard on you. Maybe, it's time for you to go somewhere else.

"We came back here because of my grandmother," she said. "Well, my grandmother has passed away now. Why don't we go someplace else before it's too late?

"I'm worried about what the Health Center is doing to you," she said. "They're giving you so many patients that you're not able to think. I think that when you were working for the health department, they were giving you patients in numbers so that if you were faced with a complicated case, you were able to think through it and come up with the right way to treat them. I think that's your true gift.

"But the way that the Health Center is throwing patients at you, there's no time for you to think. Instead, what you spend your time wrestling with after work is being traumatized by your patients or FQHC putting you down because patients don't like you.

"It's all client-based, Mike. They don't see patients as people who need responsible health care. They're customers to them. Customers whom you need to please, and I don't think that they appreciate your principled approach. It's not making their customers happy."

"I don't think that the organization is happy with you," she concluded. "I think that's what they've been trying to say in their meetings with you, especially the CEO. And they're going to keep squeezing you into their mold and getting you to do what they want.

"And with Jessica gone, there's no one to stand on your side, and they're going to keep pressing and pressing you. And I don't know if you can hold up to that sort of pressure..."

CHAPTER FORTY-EIGHT

"Mike, that doctor you knew on the Indian reservation wrote you," April said. "He said that they could hire you now, and they want you."

Hi Mike,
We spoke about a year ago about your interest in working with Native Americans and the fact that you were an NHSC Loan Repayment recipient. Did you find somewhere to fulfill your NHSC commitment? Let me know.
Best, Jim.

"Mike, Grandma's no longer here," she said. "I'm ready for a change. Before I felt a strong homing instinct to be here because my grandma was so sick. Now that she's passed – well, I have my family here, and sisters who are having babies, but, really, I don't feel the need to be here anymore, and feel ready to see something new.

"And I worried about what FQHC is doing to you. They're giving you so many patients that you're not able to think. I think that when you were working for the Health Department, they were giving you patients in numbers so that if you were faced with a complicated case, you were able to think about it, and come up with the right way to treat them. I think that's your true gift.

"But the way that FQHC is throwing patients at you, there's no time for you to think. And, instead, what you spend your time wrestling with after work is being traumatized by these patients, or FQHC putting you down because patients don't like you.

"It's all client-based, Mike. They don't see them as people who need responsible healthcare. These are customers to them.

Customers who you need to please, and I don't think they appreciate your principled stance. It's not making their customers happy.

"I don't think that the organization is happy with you. I think that's what they've been trying to say in their emails. Especially from the CEO. And they're going to keep on squeezing you into their mold, and getting you to do what they want. And with Jessica leaving, there's going to be no one to stand on your side, and the CEO is going to keep on pressing and pressing you. And I don't know if you can hold up to that sort of pressure.

"I worry about the isolation at the Indian Reservation. There would be no restaurants, no Israeli dancing, no art galleries, - none of the outlets you currently enjoy, and it might be that you'd have very little to do.

"During the night it would probably be really dark. I don't like the dark. It scares me. But, really, I've been in dark places before – like that archaeological dig in Turkey where there were only a hundred people living in that village near Diyarbakir, and, the truth is, I really liked it, because I was with so many like-minded people, and we were so into the work. I think you had that when you worked at the Health Department. I think that was really the best place for you. Because you got to take care of patients without worrying about an organization's bottom line. It was about public service. That's why I see you ultimately working for the government."

I shook my head.

I   can't,   I   said.   I've   made   a   commitment   here...

CHAPTER FORTY-NINE

Getting ready for work I cut a deep gash in my cheek while shaving.

That's funny, I thought. I've never done that before.

On the way to work I began sneezing. I'd been sneezing the night before during the Shiva service, but thought that was because April's grandma's house (where the service was held) was dusty.

Arriving at the clinic, my first patient was a woman with back pain. Accompanying her was a man in sunglasses.

"I was taking Advil and Alleve," she said, "but needed something stronger, so I went to the ER, and they gave me Hydrocodone, but I need something stronger."

There aren't many drugs stronger than Hydrocodone, I said.

Examining her, there were essentially no spasms in her back, minimal tenderness, and she demonstrated full range of motion.

"I think I heard of one in particular," she said. "It starts with a P. Purr... Purr... Percocet. Yeah, I think that's the name of it. Are you familiar with that one?"

Yes, I'm familiar with it, I said. Have you taken that medication before?

"No," she responded. "But I hear it's stronger."

Percocet has a more rapid onset of action, I said. But it isn't necessarily stronger. One of the concerning things about that medication is it's potential for addiction. Typically, I try not to prescribe it, unless there isn't another option, like patients are unable to tolerate other forms of narcotic medication.

Then, the man seated next to her interrupted.

"Didn't you say the Hydrocodone made you feel nauseous?" he said.

"Oh, yeah," she responded. "I feel nauseous."

I hesitated.

Like I said, I'd rather not prescribe you more narcotics. They have the risk of being habit forming. Where you said you'd been taking Advil and Alleve, I'd rather treat you with a stronger nonsteroidal anti-inflammatory drug like Voltaren to help with your back pain.

"I don't think I can take that one," she said. "Because I'm allergic to aspirin."

Reviewing the ER notes there had been no report of drug allergies.

"Yes, I forgot to tell them," she responded.

What reaction did you have to aspirin? I asked.

"I get a rash," she said.

Then, she looked over at the man.

"Oh, and hives," she added, tentatively. "That's it. It gives me hives."

Her response struck me as odd – like she'd been coached.

Did you have to receive medical treatment for it? I asked.

"No, because it responded to Benadryl," she said.

How long did the reaction last?

"I don't remember how long it lasted... I was young then... I can't remember the details."

"Mom took care of it," the man inserted.

"Yeah," the patient said, absently. "Right. Mom took care of it."

I turned to the man.

Are you a brother? I asked. Are the two of you related?

"No," he said. "You might say that I'm an associate."

'An associate'? I thought. What does that mean?

A urine drug screen had been performed on the patient, and showed the presence of Barbituates.

"I take them for headaches," the patient said.

Do you get them from another doctor? I asked.

"Yes," she said.

Does he treat you for your back problems, too?

"No," she said. "I just go to him for headaches."

Is he a Neurologist? I asked. Or a Headache specialist?

"No," she said. "He's primary care, like you."

Why wouldn't you ask him to treat your back pain? I thought, resisting shaking my head.

"But you said you'd been taking Advil and Alleve for your back pain, right?" I said. "Did you have any side effects with those medications?"

"No, they just didn't work as well," she responded.

I looked at the man. He remained silent and expressionless behind his sunglasses.

"It sounds like you've been able to tolerate nonsteroidal anti-inflammatory drugs, even though you're telling me you had a reaction to aspirin when you were little, though you can't be sure when," I said. "And for sure you're telling me you had a reaction to Hydrocodone since you were in the Emergency Room the other day. So, I think before I give you any more narcotics that you might react to – and, worse, potentially develop a dependence to – I'm going to try giving you this stronger form of Advil and Alleve, which haven't caused you problems. If you have any reaction, by all means, stop it, and give me a call…"

Leaving the exam room, I experienced chills and fever, and realized I was ill.

That's probably why I cut myself shaving, I thought.

Informing Lang, I requested sick leave, and went back home…

CHAPTER FIFTY

Returning to work, there was an email from the CEO sent to me and several others:

Hello everyone,
We need to schedule a sentinel event review for the patient with the above chart number who was seen today at FQHC. You are all being contacted because you as our staff had some contact with the patient's chart. The patient was seen today for back pain by one of our doctors who prescribed Voltaren for the patient's pain. The provider had documented that aspirin caused rash and hives. The patient went to our pharmacy and the medication was filled. She called FQHC when she realized that this medication was in the same class as what she is allergic to. Fortunately, because of your swift and efficient actions, she never took the medication. The front staff took the message and sent it promptly to nursing. Nursing called the patient and obtained a detailed and important medical history, including the fact that the medication was indeed filled by the pharmacy. Dr. Lang reviewed the chart and wrote for a different medication and informed the patient. We confirmed that the patient had and will not take the prescribed medication Voltaren. So although she did not take it, we need to review the case because of the potential risk if she had taken the medication...

"Why did you give the patient that medication?" April asked.

The patient had told me that she had tolerated Alleve and Advil, I said. Voltaren was another non-steroidal anti-inflammatory drug – just stronger than the others. I thought she could tolerate it, and it was better than giving her a narcotic, especially where I questioned the story of she and her 'associate' about the reaction to aspirin, and though it might be diverted to support someone's addiction or – worse – contribute to getting some young person addicted.

"Mike, they don't care that you have people's best interest at heart," she responded. "In many ways I wish you would give into the corporate culture, and for the next year and a half, give the patients the pain medications they want so the people at the clinic wouldn't be so on top of you…"

CHAPTER FIFTY-ONE

"Mike, you were sick that day, right?" April asked. "That was the day you came home early, right?... Did you tell them that?... Tell them you were sick. Tell them you weren't thinking clearly. You made that decision because you were sick. That's why you made the decision that you did. Have you ever done that before?... See? It's because you were sick! You weren't thinking straight!..."

I depressed the corners of my mouth.

I don't know, I said. Sick or not, I didn't believe her. I didn't believe she was allergic to aspirin. I thought she was coached by that fellow in the room. Maybe I would have been more self-protective, but   I   didn't   think   so...

CHAPTER FIFTY-TWO

"Mike, I looked up what a Sentinel Event is," April said. "You should take a look at the definition."

A sentinel event is any unanticipated event in a healthcare setting resulting in death or serious physical or psychological injury to a person or persons, not related to the natural course of the patient's illness.

"Mike, your patient wasn't injured," she said. "That's not what happened to her. It's all misleading.

"You have to bring up other issues, too," she continued, "like being overworked, seeing patients well into your lunch hour, and there being no effective system in place for flagging prescribed medications that patients might be allergic to?

"Mike, they give you all these patients and tell you to see them in ten minutes. They expect you to make split minute decisions based on your gut feeling. Now, they're telling you that you have to write everything down and justify every decision that you make. How are you supposed to do that? How are you supposed to do that when they're only giving you ten minutes a patient, and that includes talking to them, listening to them, examining them, requesting all the blood work, requesting all the medications, filing all the forms, ordering all the x-rays?

"Mike, you can't keep on doing this, because sooner or later you're not going to be able to shrug your shoulders and say you didn't make a mistake. One of your patients is going to have a serious reaction. And I don't think you're going to be able to live with yourself after that.

"I think that you have to act, Mike. If they want all this documentation, you have to tell them that they're forcing you to see too many patients, and bear the consequences…"

CHAPTER FIFTY-THREE

Before the Sentinel Event meeting, I pulled Lang aside, and conveyed the concerns that April and I had talked about.

"We all make more mistakes when we see higher numbers of patients," he said, blithely.

Then, he shook his head, turned and went into the conference room...

CHAPTER FIFTY-FOUR

The conference room was full; different members of the staff, starting with front office staff were called to describe their interaction with the patient. Then, it was my turn.

"Reviewing this patient's records, the patient didn't have any history of aspirin allergy in the allergy profile in the Emergency Room," I said. "In addition, she'd been to the Health Center in the past, and in all those years, she never reported any intolerances to medications on previous allergy profiles. Not until the day she met with me with this other fella in the room, who kept interrupting her with suspicious comments."

Among those present was a legal and a pain expert.

"If she did have a reaction to aspirin, why wouldn't she react to Advil or Alleve?" I directed to the experts.

"Odd," said the legal expert.

"No thoughts," said the pain expert.

Feeling a lot was riding on the decisions made here, I'd invited local DEA agent, Jack Reynolds.

"Have you considered that this patient may just be using the allergy as a false excuse for why they must have narcotics?" Reynolds posed to the group. "That the patient may have been simply drug-seeking?"

Around the table there was silence.

"We can't stop a medication she got from the ER without providing her a safe alternative," Lang asserted.

"Was what she received in the ER 'a safe alternative'?" I responded. "She described having a reaction to codeine. Was she really at less risk being prescribed a narcotic? Something habit-forming? Narcotics are medications of last resort. If you ask me, the doctor in the ER shouldn't have given the patient those medications in the first place…"

"Mike, it isn't fair to talk about the ER doctor without him here to defend himself," Lang interrupted. "It's unprofessional and inappropriate."

"But the preponderance of patients from the ER are receiving narcotics, rather than alternatives to opioids," I said.

"Mike, patients in the ER can be very forceful," he responded. "You just don't know how tough these ER providers have it, and the time constraints they're under."

"And that justifies it?" I responded. "How many patients do I see a day?... And I don't irresponsibly prescribe narcotics."

"That's because you're different," he responded.

"But why am I 'different'?" I said. "It's the same medication that we're all dealing with. A medication that causes essentially the worst side effects known to medicine – addiction and overdose. Why should we accept these 'differences'? Why wouldn't we hold these providers accountable?"

Lang smiled and sat back.

"Well, I don't think that's going to happen," he said.

"Then, let's make it happen," I responded. "Even here, I'm covering for doctors prescribing narcotics to patients with urine drug screens positive for heroin and cocaine, and negative for opiates. To protect patients and this community – as well as those physicians and this organization from the associated liability – things needs to be done."

A hush fell over the room. Lang shook his head, and turned to the CEO. The CEO glared at me, stone-faced.

"All I know," he said, "is events like this – which deliberately put our patients at risk – won't be tolerated…"

CHAPTER FIFTY-FIVE

In a holding cell I sat opposite the CEO discussing a list of patients.

"This guy admitted to using cocaine," he said. "But he still wants his dose of narcotics upped, OK?"

I nodded, and then was escorted out of the holding cell. I was being let out of the prison on good behavior to work at the clinic.

Why doesn't he get one of his other goons to prescribe this? I thought, as I made my way down the fenced-enclosed path to the outside.

OK, I thought, I'll do it. But I won't prescribe the narcotics myself. I'll refer the patient to pain management...

Awakening from the dream, I couldn't believe how real it seemed.

"Yeah," April said. "It's too bad they now have this case to hold against you..."

CHAPTER FIFTY-SIX

"You're not diplomatic," April continued. "Instead of saying something to diffuse the situation, you're setting them off. It's not like it's going to impact patient care. Like it's going to be bad for the patient. Just say, 'OK, you're the boss.' It's not like he's asking you to do something illegal or bad for the patient. Just eat shit a little bit. Say, 'I'll do it.' Smooth things over, so you can move on to something else. Because they're just going to get to the point where they say, 'I just can't deal with him anymore.' And then they're going to break you. And all that can be avoided if you just say, 'Sure, fine.'"

"The other doctors are doing it," she continued. "I think it's just because you're such a rigid person. You get on a high horse sometimes, and there's no getting you off of it."

She shook his head.

"I'm trying to tell you how to handle this," she said. "Don't make it into a professional issue with you. In order to get rid of you, they won't say, 'We just couldn't get along.' They're going to say you're a bad doctor. They don't mind destroying somebody's career. Life. You don't have Jessica to protect you anymore. She's out. She isn't here to tell the CEO, 'Let go of it. It's OK.'"

"Smooth it over," she pleaded. "For our sake. I'm telling you, if you don't make some changes, our days here are numbered..."

Letter to the CEO:

This letter is in reference to the Sentinel Event that occurred. The purpose of the meeting was in regards to the performance deficiency of the doctor involved. Even before the meeting I got the impression that he is overwhelmed as a clinician. He does 'shotgun' treatment as shown in the Sentinel Event. More extensive chart reviews are needed to correct these deficiencies. I recommend more oversight in the form of shadowing or precepted sessions to get him to that level of competency that FQHC requires.

Sincerely,
Bradley Lang...

CHAPTER FIFTY-SEVEN

April read the letter.

"'Not up to FQHC standards,'" she said. "And what are those 'standards'? Not handing out enough narcotics? Mike, what did you say to him when he made comments like these?"

When I'd received the notice, I tried to pull Lang aside. But he just shook his head, waved me off and walked away.

"But don't you feel like you have to respond to this?" she said. "Why don't you stand up for yourself?"

When someone points a finger at you, they point four at themselves, I said. Considering the source, I didn't think it merits much more of a response. I just want to get back to work, and let that do the talking for me.

"I don't know," she said. "I see you get hunched, and quiet, and let him do and say to you whatever he wants. Is this a pattern with you? When you were a kid, did you let your mom and dad treat you this way?"

Perhaps, I said. When they'd act irrationally, I'd usually just wait it out. Indeed, when they took things out on me, I just took it, in hopes that they'd feel bad about it, and get over it quicker.

"Mike, standing down or walking away or not saying anything to someone whose being irrational is one thing. But this isn't about people being irrational. This is about people taking advantage of you. And I don't see where you're fighting back. When someone criticizes me, I immediately defend myself. But you haven't been doing that."

I sighed.

"If you ask me," I said, "the fact that they're taking actions like this I believe is more a blemish on their record than mine. This is no way to treat someone devoted to public service, and with as much to lose as I have – and they know it…"

CHAPTER FIFTY-EIGHT

"What ultimately happened with the patient?" April asked. "The one they called the Sentinel Event for."

Lang immediately prescribed narcotics for her, I said. But repeated urine drug screens showed there were no opiates in her system, suggesting they were being diverted.

I'd actually seen the patient the day before. Standing at the door I took a deep breath, envisioning the conversation to come. Then, stepping into the examination room, I was surprised to find two small boys as well as the patient. Neither of the children could have been more than five years old. I felt nauseous. How am I supposed to say what I have with these children here?

Somehow, though, the visit commenced.

"What do you think I'm here for?" the patient said. "Just to look at your pretty face? I need the pain-killers for the pain in my back. The other medicines make me break out in hives."

The children in the chair began to fidget and bicker.

"Scoot over," one boy said. "You have more room."

"No, you do," the other responded.

The patient hushed the children; the boys responded with stunning obedience, pulling themselves upright, and not uttering another word.

I held firm that the narcotic pain pills could not be continued. As the visit drew to a close, the children asked if they could have some stickers? Searching the drawers, I found some colored Band-Aids, and distributed them to the boys, who cheered with glee.

You talk about putting a Band-Aid on a gushing wound, I thought...

"Don't feel sorry for these patients, Mike!" April responded. "Most of the stories that they're telling you are lies!"

"They are taking away your time!" she continued. "When they do that, they take away health! They take away life, because they're keeping you from helping patients who need you, who are poor and have no other place to go and can really use your services — to say nothing of the toll that it exacts from you every day!"

I nodded, but really my thoughts are elsewhere: Back with those two little boys walking in tow behind their mother, happily carrying those colored Band-Aids into an uncertain future...

To: Michael Kadima, MD

From: Bradley Lang, MD

Re: Notice of Performance Deficiency

cc: Personnel file

Since you began work at FQHC, your work performance has not meet FQHC standards and this has resulted in a number of performance deficiencies including substandard clinical management for potentially life-threatening medical concerns by prescribing medication for a patient to which she had a documented allergy to medication in a similar class.

In reviewing your charts over the past 9 months we have noted a similar type of performance deficiency: Patient prescribed azithromycin (a macrolide) for respiratory infection. It was prescribed despite the documentation of an allergy to erythromycin (also a macrolide).

Your work performance does not meet FQHC standards and this has resulted in a number of patient and staff complaints. Please note that your contract specifies the following: 'FQHC may immediately terminate your employment if you fail or refuse to perform your duties to FQHC's general satisfaction, or otherwise breach any provision of the contract.'

Specific remediation includes achieving 100% compliance with FQHC's expectation for documentation in history of present illness, physical examination, assessment and treatment section in the chart.

Please consider this letter of reprimand to be formal notice of your performance deficiencies. You have 30 days to remedy these issues…

CHAPTER FIFTY-NINE

I went to Lang to discuss the Azithromycin case cited in the reprimand, reminding him that although in the same 'family' as Erythromycin, it rarely caused stomach upset.

"Do you know that?" he said. "Can you be sure of that?"

Yes, I responded. The patient had no side effects with the Azithromycin. He'd actually taken it before. I'd asked him before prescribing the medication.

He shook his head.

"The patient had an allergic reaction to Erythromycin, and you gave the patient something in the same family," he remarked, sarcastically. "Shotgun medicine..."

"Mike, they're just looking for things to reprimand you," April said. "This man isn't your friend. That's his name on that reprimand. You don't have Jessica anymore to protect you. You should just quit that job while you still can. Do you think you're going to have an easy job getting another when they terminate you?"

"Mike, they're using scare tactics," April said. "'We can fire you.' You know what they're doing – they're combing the carts looking for mistakes to back them up. They're not looking at the good things you do.

"Mike, if you can't support kids financially, and I can't support them, then we can't have them. I know this is affecting you more than me, and you're doing the best you can. What can I say?"

She put her hands to her head.

"Mike, why doesn't the FQHC just tell you why they don't want you?" she said. "Why are they planning all this time combing through your charts trying to find something when really they've known for months why they don't want you? They're just not telling you. They're keeping it behind your back. They're being tricky. They have the reason that they don't want you, but they're just not telling you. They just won't tell you.

"I think that if you were dealing with Jessica, she'd just tell you straight off, 'The FQHC just doesn't want you.' I can't believe that this would be happening on her watch. But the FQHC won't do that. Instead, they're trying to find an excuse."

She shook her head.

"Mike, I want you out of this job," she said. "I have been ready for a while for you to quit that job because you are not able to be the doctor that you're meant to be. This is not the right fit for you.

"They're a pill mill, Mike," she continued, "and they're just going to get worse, because to them it's too expensive to do anything else. Their moto is, 'If people want to kill themselves and send themselves into oblivion, more money for us. They're just making themselves into prey, and we like prey. Because they're weak, and they're not going to do anything about that. And if we can make money off of it. That's good for us.'

"Mike, they're saying 100%. That's not reasonable, Mike. They're not being reasonable. Don't you know what that means? They're talking to you that way because they don't want you around. They don't want you there, Mike. It's loud and clear. They're not interested in improvement. They're not interesting in helping you to fix a problem. They just want you out.

"It's loud and clear. That's what they're saying, and that's what they're gonna do. You should get on the phone and call the Reservation and let them know that you're interested. And if they're interested, then take that job, and quit this job before they fire you, and permanently damage your medical career..."

CHAPTER SIXTY

Investigating a hideous crime that took place within a prison, I was going in and out of the quarantined area by scaling fences. There were three places I could go: Within the quarantine area; outside the quarantine area, and the space in between.

Walking in the alley between the fences, a voice called to me: "You don't have to be there anymore."

"Yeah, but I can think here," I responded.

I'd been traversing the fences when the stony faced FQHC CEO came and shook at fence till I went falling off.

Striking the ground, I awoke from the dream.

Sitting up, I nodded.

I'm in prison, I thought. It's by my own choice – because there's still good work to be done in between.

I went to my computer.

Jessica, I feel the need to write you about recent happenings at FQHC...

Hi Michael,

I hate being so far over here from all of you. I read about the Sentinel Event because Brad sent it to me to review. I said that the case was very difficult as there are no records about previous aspirin allergy. I think you documented her comments well, but it did seem that from front to back there were issues.

Thanks for your time.

Jessica...

CHAPTER SIXTY-ONE

Given an assignment to train in flight for crop dusting, I was feeling nervous; people were standing atop the wings doing acrobatics as I flew. What if I hit a tree? I thought. What if I had to make a difficult landing? What if these people got hurt? I was afraid that I didn't have the ability to balance all these people.

I called Jessica, told her about the assignment, and asked if she had any interest in training with me?

"No," she responded. "I can't..."

Awakening from the dream, I reflected on Jessica's absence; how she was no longer at FQHC to support me; and no matter how hard I worked, without a source of support in the clinic, patients were in danger.

I remembered the letter we'd composed to the CEO; the one about the patient who'd been treated with Suboxone, then refused to provide a medical release, so I could talk with his doctors.

I'd been her foil, I thought. I was the one who'd say the things she wanted – Take the stands she wanted. Now, she was on the outside.

Still, she's training young physicians to enter primary care. Is FQHC a place she wants them? Facing the kind of adversity I am?...

Michael,

I do not recollect these conversations with you, and I had quite a different experience. A lot of the standardized care we had at FQHC meets disease core measures. I am not saying your experience is not different, but I honestly felt I provided good care and our work was above and beyond what I have seen elsewhere.

To answer of your question- yes I feel comfortable. Two of my residents have graduated here and will be practicing there soon. Are there some residents I might not send there? Absolutely but for a variety of reasons. Honestly, many of us struggle in practice at other places, too. FQHC has pharmacy, med assistance programs, psych, gyn, dental, diabetes educators all on site which is so much better than just being a doc on your own. No?

I realize your time at FQHC has not been ideal. You and I have both worked other places, for whatever reason this is not a good fit for you and that is unfortunate since you enjoy the state and family you have nearby.

Jessica...

CHAPTER SIXTY-TWO

"Of course, she wasn't going to speak against FQHC," April said. "She was the previous Clinical Director there. Now, you've jeopardized her being a reference for you…"

CHAPTER SIXTY-THREE

As I was about to go to the clinic's Thanksgiving party, when I was called to attend a patient. She came for refills of narcotic medication; however, she was tachycardic, with a heart rate of 152, widely dilated pupils, and review of the medical record indicated she had a recent history of cocaine use. But when I asked her about recent use, she denied it. The nurse supervisor intervened.

"All she wants is her pain medication," she said.

But I didn't feel comfortable, especially as each passing moment, the patient's heart rate kept climbing. I recommended ER transfer, but the patient refused.

The nursing supervisor was incensed.

"Her heart is beating that way because she's angry about not being given her meds!" she declared loudly…

"That's the problem," April said. "They just want you to get the patients in and out of there. Who cares that her heart is beating a mile a minute and she's probably high on cocaine. It's your job to move the patients…"

Provider Progress Report.

Patient seen by you for refill of Hydrocodone states that she had to go to the Emergency Department for medication. Patient states that you would not give her medication refill because she's had incidents with cocaine, but says she is not using now. She feels asking her to give a urine sample is disrespectful. She feels that she needs to be treated with respect at all visits and should not have to give a urine sample and would like another provider.

I did note the abnormal utox screen, but did not tell the patient.

Patient transferred to locums while await your 30-day evaluation following official reprimand.

Bradley Lang...

CHAPTER SIXTY-FOUR

Over Shabbat dinner with her parents, April shared the difficulties at FQHC. Her mother expressed surprise.

"Wasn't your CEO the one we met at the Wesleyan Pottery?" she asked. "The person I remember was young and idealistic, just like you. I thought that the two of you were a natural fit together. Do you think that you can write him, and explain the situation?"

April interrupted.

"Mom, that organization is an extension of him," April said. "It's no accident that he's the watchdog over that organization to come after anyone who strays from their way of doing things."

"Yeah, I know," she said. "But what if we look at things from their view. You said they wrote that staff worried about him - that they didn't like the way he did things and were reporting back about that. What if they have a legitimate concern? What if it wasn't about you not giving out enough narcotics and tests and referrals and disability, but instead that they were really worried about patients being harmed? And all the CEO had to go by was what the staff told him because he wasn't hearing anything from you? Don't you think that it would be better if he got your side of the story?"

"It's too late for that, mom," April said. "Mike's already talked to him, and they're still taking action against him."

April turned to her father.

"Dad, if Mike goes into default with the NHSC, can that debt fall on me?" April asked.

"I don't know," he said. "You need to ask a lawyer."

"Because it's a large debt, and I've been looking for whether there's any way around it. Like a prenuptial agreement, though it seems a little late for that."

"I don't know," he said. "Like I told you, I think that those are questions for a lawyer."

"April, what are you talking about?" I said. "'Prenuptial agreements'? We have to fight this thing, not dream up ways to get around it."

"But I don't think you can win," she said. "You've been fighting it for the past year, and haven't got anywhere – except made a lot of people mad. You're in the gears of a big bureaucracy, Mike, and they're going to do and say anything they want. It's just like the FQHC. They've lined things up against you. The NHSC will do the same thing."

"April, if the worst happens, and FQHC lets go of me, I'll work at another NHSC site," I said.

"That's what you say, but they can do whatever they want with you," she said.

"You are so negative," I retorted. "You are just so negative."

I shook my head.

"Where does this come from?" I continued. "Where does this attitude of 'I can't' come from with you? This isn't the way you go into battle. 'I can't.' 'I can't.' 'I can't.' You have to fight for what you can do."

"Guys, don't argue," Doris said. "Not on Shabbat."

Gazing up at my father-in-law, he was looking at me with wide-eyed, obviously at a loss for words.

Leaving, Doris didn't offer her usual hug...

CHAPTER SIXTY-FIVE

April found a lawyer. We met with him in the evening at his downtown office.

"Mike, where did you work before this?" he asked.

The Tennessee Health Department, I said. At a community medical center that also served as a satellite clinic of the VA.

"Then, you're used to the kind of cases that come through the FQHC's door, right?" he said. "Mike, besides the problem of giving medicine to patients with allergies, what else have patients complained about?"

Narcotic prescribing, I responded.

He nodded.

"Mike, around the time that these things happened, was there anything happening in your life that might have distracted you from work?"

I shook my head, but April intervened.

"Around the time that these things happened," she said, "my grandmother was dying, and I was very needy, and leaning on Mike for personal support, and think that could have affected Mike's performance on the job."

"What do you think about that, Mike?" the lawyer asked. "Do you think it affected you?"

I thought about running that razor across my cheek, and the gouge it left on my skin.

"I really don't like to make excuses," I said.

"Mike, let me tell you something," he said. "I got into some trouble once. My father was sixty, and diagnosed with prostate cancer. I went through a time where everything was coming down on me and really didn't know what to do, and it crept into my work. But these things happened to people, Mike."

I depressed the corners of my mouth and shrugged.

"I mean, what do you think?" he continued. "Do you like the work you're doing?"

My thoughts drifted to my drug seeking patients.

"Mike, it just doesn't sound like this is the right place for you," he said. "And what I see in here is a really good, caring doctor who just needs to be someplace else."

He lifted the FQHC deficiency notices.

"Look, Mike, I've read through your stuff, and I don't see any glaring issues here," he said. "No one ever got hurt, and the reviews are just picking on a lot of petty stuff."

I'd shared my email correspondence with Jessica.

"Mike, what's your relationship with this doctor you wrote to?" he asked. "You said she was your previous Clinical Director, right?... Well, maybe you and I can construct an email so she says that you're doing a good job. That could be an important bit of evidence if this ever goes to court."

I shook my head, saying I didn't want to manipulate Jessica.

"Well, what do you want to do, Mike?" he asked.

I want to tell them, Don't do this, have some faith, keep the discussion going, don't stop, I want to keep working, and don't want to give up.

He shook his head.

"Mike, you don't want to do this. It doesn't sound to me like you deserve what they're doing to you. You haven't shown up at work intoxicated. You don't drink on the job. You haven't taken narcotics. You haven't done anything criminal.

"Just looking at you, Mike, it doesn't look like you're doing very well. You look tense. You don't look happy.

"So, I'll talk to them, and say that I think you're a very upstanding, moral doctor, and try to work it out.

"Keep in mind, though, if they do terminate you, there's nothing you can do about it. You signed an 'at-will' contract in a 'right-to-work' state. They can let you go whenever they want.

"The problem, of course, is when you're a medical professional, and the workplace complains about you, it can be hard to get another job. Other employers tend to just go along with the word of your previous employer if you get into trouble. And if they can claim they fired you because of your medical judgment, well, anytime there's the appearance of anything like that, essentially nobody will touch you. I've represented docs who've essentially lost their careers in medicine

as a result...”

CHAPTER SIXTY-SIX

It didn't seem right, I thought, leaving the lawyer's office. Treating physicians this way. Physicians who wish to serve their country; who sign up for the NHSC; and are then threatened with termination and default just because they're trying to be responsible clinicians.

"This is why I stopped being religious as a kid," April responded. "It's because I got really mad at God."

"You're all about 'standing before God,'" she continued, "and being able to say that you 'did your best.' That you 'lived a good life.' That you were 'honest.'

"But, Mike, you do live in the world. You do live in the physical plain. You do need to protect yourself.

"Because that's life in the physical plain. You have to protect yourself. And that's just not in you, Mike. That's why you have to let me and Simon help you. It's just not in you to protect yourself. You don't know how to do it.

"You think life is all about goodness, but, look, in this world, how do creatures survive? How do you survive? You survive by eating other living things. The only creature that doesn't live off another are plants and algae. They use photosynthesis. And even they have defenses against others so that they can claim the territory that they need to live.

"In this world, Mike, it's eat or be eaten. You won't survive by telling the truth. By being good all the time. That's naïve. You have to protect yourself, and you haven't done that. You've relied on others to see your goodness and judge you because you're earnest. And they didn't care anything about that. They just wanted you to fit into their model. And if you weren't going to do that, then they were going to take you out.

"You were all worried about being accused of fraud if you ordered too many tests, or that it would be irresponsible and subtract from more patients being able to get healthcare that you were trying to bolster. And you were worried about giving out too many pain pills because it was causing problems in the community. And your employers don't care anything about that. What they care about is making patients happy, and you aren't doing that, and they're going to take you out. It's eat or be eaten, Mike. You understand that. You're being eaten.

"And in this eat or be eaten world, humans are the worst predators, because they kill more than they can eat. And they kill for other reasons, too..."

CHAPTER SIXTY-SEVEN

April sat at the kitchen table putting figures into a calculator.

"I've done the calculations," she said. "If you resign and the NHSC puts you in default, the best that we can hope for is to be asked to pay back $133,000. This is contingent on the NHSC accepting the six months that you worked for FQHC. If the NHSC does not credit the six months you worked there because you didn't finish, then you could wind up in default for $200,000 plus the highest interest allowable by law beginning from when you began there. If after seven years, you're not able to pay all of it, you can declare bankruptcy. The problem is, once they put you in default, you'll never be able to charge the Centers of Medicare and Medicaid for patient services. And you won't be able to take a job with the federal government, so you'll never work for the VA again..."

CHAPTER SIXTY-EIGHT

At the end of the week I got off work too late to welcome Shabbat with April's family. Still, they put aside some food, and kept me company around the table.

"Well, I appreciate your efforts to keep April here during my mother's last months," Doris said, "and had to work very hard in this bureaucratic place that hasn't appreciated what you've had to give."

"Other places, the doctor is king," April said. "That isn't always a good thing. But at FQHC, the doctors are treated like shit, and completely held accountable to the will of the patients. With FQHC, the patient calls all the shots. And if you don't do what the patient wants, you're out of there."

Doris showed me a flier.

"I got this flier from the local high school," she said. "Tonight they're sponsoring a performance. It's featuring Elisabeth Von Trapp."

Von Trapp, I thought. That name sounds familiar? Where have I heard that name before?

"Her grandmother was Maria Von Trapp, whose life was the basis for 'The Sound of Music,'" Doris said. "She was the nun who leaves the convent to become a governess, and then marries that captain with all those children."

That was a true story? I said. I thought it was made up.

"No, they're real people," she responded. "After the Von Trapps left Austria because of the Nazis, they emigrated to the United States and settled in Vermont. It says that Elizabeth Von Trapp performs mostly folk songs about growing up there. You want to go to the concert?"

I shook my head. I wasn't much in the mood for musicals. Really, I wasn't in the mood for anything.

"Come on, Mike," April said. "You'll like it. It will be fun..."

The event was sponsored by the Creative Living Community, which provides services for adults diagnosed with autism and developmental disabilities.

As the event began, Ms. Von Trapp took the stage. Looking at her, it was hard not to be struck by her uncanny resemblance to Julie Andrews, who played her grandmother in the movie that earned her an Oscar.

Ms. Von Trapp performed several original works, but really shined when she sang the songs her grandmother inspired.

As she sang *My Favorite Things* those all around me seemed incapable of restraining themselves from swaying side-to-side and singing along with child-like glee.

Raindrops on roses and whiskers on kittens,
Bright copper kettles and warm woolen mittens,
Brown paper packages tied up with strings,
These are a few of my favorite things.

Then, in a soaring rendering of *Climb Every Mountain* Ms. Von Trapp seemed to channel the Reverend Mother who sent her grandmother on her life's journey more than 50 years ago.

Climb every mountain, search high and low.
Follow every byway, every path you know.
Climb every mountain, ford every stream.
Follow every rainbow, 'til you find your dream.

April nestled me.

"It's about love, Mike," she whispered. "It's about love."

No, it's not, I scowled. It's about pills. It's about tests. It's about clients. It's about having a job, and then doing whatever it takes to keep that job. Because if you lose that job, who knows what's going to happen.

Looking about at the school children in attendance, I felt a deep ache in my chest.

What is there for these children? I thought. Once I felt a sense of purpose. A willingness to surrender to love and the calling of my heart. What was there to live for now?

Just then, Ms. Von Trapp interrupted her performance to address the audience.

"Now, I'd like to take this opportunity to invite a very special young man to perform," she says. "His name is Karl, and he's going to accompany me on the cello."

Karl is 19, and has autism. He did not speak until he was 4, but had a gift for music, and at age 5 began playing the cello, and has excelled in performing with that instrument ever since. He plays beautifully.

"Now, Karl is going to accompany me on a duet," Ms. Von Trapp continues. "And I can't think of anyone else with whom I'd rather sing this song."

The two begin to sing:

When you wish upon a star,
Makes no difference who you are,
Anything your heart desires
Will come to you.

And as those in attendance got to their feet to embrace this young man with a standing ovation, I rose, too...

CHAPTER SIXTY-NINE

FQHC, INC. NEW CONSTRUCTION TO BEGIN.
This is extremely exciting!...

During the week I was moved from one cubicle to another on two separate occasions, each closer to the new construction, so that the sound of jackhammers around me felt like they were drilling into my head.

"It's Holocaust Remembrance Day," Doris announced over Shabbat dinner. "There's a concert featuring music composed at the Terezin Ghetto. That where our family was interned before sent to the death camps. None of the composers survived the Holocaust. Are you interested in going?"

I'd been making plans to attend a Grateful Dead concert, where I was looking to drown my persistent headache by losing myself in their melodies. And the tickets for the Terezin music were not inexpensive.

Seems like a lot of money for a depressing evening, I thought.

But I couldn't shake the feeling like I had to do something to observe the Remembrance Day...

The event was held in a church, and scanning those in attendance, it didn't seem like there were many Jewish faces. Certainly, the performers weren't Jewish. The singer was Swedish. The violinist English. What did they know about the Holocaust experience?

The opening compositions were haunting, and spoke to feelings of sadness, hopelessness and desperation. When the intermission came, I greeted it with relief.

Doris was moved.

"It makes me feel good to know that if the members of my family had to be in that dreadful place, at least they had music," she said.

As the music resumed, it felt as though I were teleported to the ghetto, and with each score I felt more and more connected with the fate of my long departed brethren; as if I were right there with them, trapped in the ghetto, then riding in those transport trains to the death camps (mostly Auschwitz).

Line me up, and shoot me where I stand, I thought. Or put me into a gas chamber, and then burn my flesh to ashes. But, God in Your mercy, give me the courage to live a righteous life.

And then, when all seemed lost and no hope left, the concert ended. Those in attendance stood and applauded.

And I stood, too - but it was mostly to acknowledge those all around me who cared enough to honor the murdered composers, so that their works could endure, their cause remembered, and their spirit saved for the ages...

CHAPTER SEVENTY

Arriving at the Health Center, my medical assistant asked if I would be away for the week?

"Because according to the schedule, you have several days off," she said.

I asked Brad.

"I don't know where it's coming from," he said, nonchalantly, and walked past.

I wrote to the CEO. No response.

Then, lo-and-behold, my schedule opened, and I was seeing patients.

When I called April at lunch, she was excited.

"All your hard work paid off," she said.

Then, one of the first patients from when I started working – the one who I diagnosed with early stage lung cancer – came for an appointment.

"I'm need a refill of my pain medicine," he told me. "I'm still having chest pain from where they did the surgery."

He'd been receiving a narcotic medication. But, on the urine drug screen, he tested negative for it.

I looked at him surprised.

"You said you took the last pill yesterday," I said. "It isn't showing up in your system."

He smiled.

"Well, maybe I took the last one the day before," he responded.

"Even if you'd taken it the day before, you should test positive for it," I said.

"Well," he said, still smiling, "does that mean you're not going to give me it?"

"I can't justify it," I said. "Really, you shouldn't be out of it. You were prescribed enough to still have some till the end of the week."

He continued, smiling, as he made his way out of the exam room.

A few minutes later I got an email from Nancy in Human Resources.

Please call at your convenience.

I decided to put patients first, and decided to wait until I had a break, so I wouldn't keep patients waiting.

Then, an email came from the CEO.

You need to call Nancy.

I called her.

"Thank you for calling," she stuttered. "I appreciate you getting back to me. What I want to say is, don't come into the clinic until we've resolved the issue of the chart reviews. We're still working on that and should come to some decision soon."

It left me stunned.

Why hadn't she just written that? I thought.

I wrote to the CEO, informing him of the discussion.

You need you to do what Marcia says. This is not vacation or paid time off. Don't tell others. They can't help you.

I looked at the computer screen; the names of my patients on my schedule were deleted before my eyes. The hepatitis patient who needed a liver transplant. The patient who'd just been diagnosed with HIV and needed treatment. The tuberculosis patient who'd just been found to have a lytic lesion in his spine. All those names dwindling before my eyes. There'd initially been 36 patients scheduled for me tomorrow. Now that number was 12. When I looked again, it was 10.

"They've made their decision," April said.

The number fell to 8, then 7.

I turned away from the computer at five.

I informed my medical assistant. She looked down.

"I hope they'll let you stay," she said. "The patients are very difficult. There is so little time. We were doing our best…"

CHAPTER SEVENTY-ONE

"They weren't happy with you, Mike," April said. "You weren't doing things their way. They wanted to get rid of you, and didn't matter how hard you work. Because sometimes it is a matter of how hard you work – it's about, how you work. And you weren't working their way. They were going to do everything in their power to discredit you.

"Look at what happened to you. Look at how they organized things. That sentinel review. They organize a public forum just to humiliate you in front of your coworkers. That was no sentinel review. That was no reportable case. It was something where you should have been asked the question, 'Why did you prescribe that medication?' Instead they made it this whole public forum to humiliate you.

"Look at the timing, Mike. What does the CEO wait for before sending the deficiency letter? He waits for Jessica – the lioness – to be out of the picture. But, in the end, even when she was out of there, she wouldn't stand up to him.

"Think about it, Mike. Where was Brad when you were moved from that one pod to another. Jessica wasn't there. So, he was the acting Medical Director, right? Did he say anything? Did he stop what was going on?... No. He'd made his feelings known to you before. 'Make the patients happy, or else they'll make life hell for you.'

"Mike, Brad is totally dependent on the CEO. He's unsure of himself. You remember that letter he wrote? Well in advance of what happened, he communicated with you that he wasn't protecting you. He told you. He had been straightforward with you that he was not standing in the CEO's way. He told you that he wasn't going to be an

135

advocate. He was actually being harsher on you on an official level than the other people were. And then he stayed away from you. He betrayed you in the sense that he didn't fight for you. But he did not betray you in the sense that he didn't communicate to you where he stood. He was loud and clear in that letter that he wasn't going to stand behind you. That he would let you be beset upon.

"You were being very hard-headed in wanting to believe that hard work would change their minds. The writing was on the wall. They were communicating – well, not really. They were giving you indirect messages – that I was getting – that they were letting you go. But in the paperwork they were looking like they were giving you a chance. And you were grasping at that. But they were giving you a lot of signals that they weren't really giving you a chance.

"I mean, come on, they prepared that deficiency letter a month before they gave it to you, and then when they gave it to you, they gave you an evening to review it! No good faith there. No attempt to see your side of it. That's people who have given up.

"And you were being very un-self-protective. It comes from your experience at Aaron County, but different situations are different. You can't always go by what happened in the past, because with this it's different sorts of people. Maybe you can, but I'd say you should have fought for a different job, instead of fighting for this job, and you would have lost a position, but you would have tried to get out – you would have given FQHC the chance to not destroy you.
"But you didn't. The only choice you gave them was to continue to swallow what they didn't like about you. You were thinking that they didn't have the ruthlessness to destroy you – you gave it your all, but they were not being receptive anymore.

"You never had a chance there. The concerns that you were addressing – the things that you were trying to do better – those weren't the real things that they wanted you to change. It wasn't about your documentations or the tests you ordered. It was about patient complaints. They were complaining about you, and that was leaving the clinic rattled. They wanted someone who could smooth over complaints – who could tell a patient no that would leave that person placated, or who would just give patients the medications to pacify them – or the disability, or the referrals. And you weren't going to do that.

"So they found other things to attack you with. You worked your hardest, Mike, to do things better and make improvements the way that said. You treated them with good faith, and for the past month, the FQHC has been your whole life.

"But they were never going to give you a chance, Mike. Can't you see?..."

CHAPTER SEVENTY-TWO

April had been seeing a therapist since her grandmother's passing, and suggested I accompany her to an appointment.

"For the past months I've watched as this fun loving man," April said, "who loves flowers and loves children - this man has disappeared into work and stress. I've wanted him to give up this job since September. I could see the writing on the wall since then. But Mike wanted to work with them. He wanted to work through these things. So, I'm happy now that it looks like this thing is going to be over."

The therapist turned to me.

"Mike, what was the hook that really brought you into this group?" the therapist asked.

They told me they were about transparency, I said, working thru problems, getting past setbacks, bringing out the best that the best minds had to offer.

"The corporate world doesn't always work very well, and success looks different to them," the therapist responded. "'Patients who are happy,' not healthy. But their demands are that you do it their way, and that didn't work for you."

"But they couldn't control Mike," April inserted. "Couldn't bully him, so they had to let him go."

"Yes, they have the power," the therapist said. "Which is too bad for them that they didn't see the good in Mike."

She sat back.

"It sounds like, where your patients were concerned, they'd given up on them, too," she said. "'Just make them happy' – that doesn't sound like a very good formula for making patients well. You'd be giving up on them if you just gave them drugs. You were trying to get your patients to a place where they can be more than they are, and to be able to do that in the constraints of this job – with 20 patients a day – is really remarkable, laudable and should have been rewarded. Instead, you're punished, which doesn't make sense, but that she upside down world we live in – there's nothing that you can do about that. You just have to get used to it, and deal with it, and find the right place for you."

"The problem with Mike is that he's not always practical," April said. "I'll give you an example. Usually, we take walks in a nearby park that has something called 'Rails for Trails.' But as winter was approaching, it was getting darker sooner. But Mike was under so much stress, and I felt like the walk was helping him, so against my better judgment, I went along when he wanted to walk longer. And it did get dark, and I was really scared on the walk back, especially when I thought I heard a snake on the trail. So, I'm less trusting of Mike's judgment, because I don't feel like he always does things to protect himself..."

CHAPTER SEVENTY-THREE

"Mike, if you could tell these people what you really felt, and you didn't have this NHSC thing on your back, what would you tell them?" the therapist asked.

I'd say, This is no way to treat people, and if you're going to persist, I'm going to have to go elsewhere.

"What's keeping you from saying that?"

Because it was all there, I responded. If they'd just been willing to work with me, we could have accomplished so much.

"Were you willing to work with them?"

Yes. I was spending countless hours working. I was the first in in the morning, and the last to leave at night. I wanted to learn from the changes that they were suggesting.

"So you were doing all you could, and it still wasn't enough for them."

I stared up; April had said that I was duped from the beginning, and the writing was on the wall from the start that they weren't looking to work with me. I felt like, if I had lived during the Holocaust, I would have wound up letting the Nazis march me right to the gas chambers, because I was going to keep on 'working with them, and waiting for them to come around to their senses.

"In this case," the therapist said, "it sounds like April was right, and they weren't going to work with you..."

CHAPTER SEVENTY-FOUR

"FQHC is sowing the seeds of their own destruction," the therapist continued. "Perhaps not at this time, but someday they'll pay for their mistake of losing you. From everything April's told me, you go the extra mile in taking care of others. What you don't seem to focus on is taking care of yourself.

"You're better off getting away from this group. You didn't deserve this. You didn't do anything wrong. Put yourself first – and leave this group. Do what's best for you and April, and let go of this job."

"You did what you could to get them to behave responsibly, and that's all you could do," she concluded. "You kept your end of the bargain. That's why you can move on with your head held high..."

CHAPTER SEVENTY-FIVE

At the house I was packing when I heard my mother shouting and stomping through the house. Then, when it seemed she was nearly upon me - her anger intensified - I threw myself upon the suitcase, and stood paralyzed, like I couldn't move, and just had to sit there and take it.

Awakening from the dream, I thought about yesterday's conversation with April's therapist – and how it was that when people pushed against me, I had a tendency to accept it, and just take it. And that was the pattern with my mother.

"Why would you do that?" April said.

Because she was my mother. There was really no place to go. And after beating up on me, she would usually cool down, and then regret it – and I could get back to what was important, which was completing my schoolwork. And who knows? Maybe my letting her beat up on me might have helped relieve her tension, and this was my way of giving back to her, because I did appreciate her taking care of me. After all, she was my protector.

"That's what you tried to do with FQHC," April said. "Only they didn't feel any personal loyalty to you – like your mother – and the first chance they could get, they were going to push you out…"

CHAPTER SEVENTY-SIX

April got a call from her mom that an elderly relation named Hanne was being taken to the Emergency Room.

"She has a bad infection in her leg," Doris said. "She said that she hurt her leg a couple of days ago. Her caregiver thinks that she must have bumped into a table while she was getting around in her wheelchair, and took off some of the skin."

"Do you know Hanne's story?" my mother-in-law continued. "Well, since my mother died, Hanne is the sole surviving member of the family who lived through the Holocaust. Her life was somewhat like Anne Frank's. She grew up a hidden child. I think you'd find her story interesting…"

We met Hanne and her caregiver at the Emergency Room lobby.

"The wound is all red and swollen," the caregiver said. "I asked Hanne if she told anyone about it, but she said that she didn't want to be a bother, and that's why she hadn't said anything before."

"It's just a scratch," Hanne insisted. "I didn't want to waste your time over it."

"I called her doctor," the caregiver continued, "and he was insistent that I take Hanne to the hospital to get the wound looked at. I examined the wound. It was inflamed and tender, and I felt sad that I hadn't been told about it earlier, so I could come by and offer treatment before this."

"This was the first time that I've been to Hanne's in three months," the caregiver continued. "It was only because her other caregiver, Annie, went to visit her mother for Christmas. Annie doesn't have any medical training or experience, so I imagine that's why she didn't notice the wound or give it much thought. I guess it was just lucky that I was around to see it."

The caregiver smiled broadly.

"Everything happens for a reason," the caregiver said, cheerfully. "That's what I always say."

Listening, I couldn't help but wonder what Hanne thought of her caregiver's statement, seeing that Hanne had lived through one of the worst periods in human history?...

CHAPTER SEVENTY-SEVEN

"Well, I have to leave now," the caregiver said. "I have some clients at a group home that I have to check in on. I'll call tomorrow to see how things went here."

The caregiver departed, and we waited with Hanne in the emergency room.

"I'm sorry that you felt like you needed to come out here," Hanne said. "It's really nothing. I'm sure that it will get better on its own."

After blood work was performed, April suggested I go to the gym and work out.

"Yes, go," Hanne said. "Have fun."

Maybe that was a good idea, I thought, as I hadn't exercised in a while.

But, rising to my feet, I realized that, really, I didn't want to leave.

"I'm a sucker for a good story," I told Hanne. "And from what I understand, you've had an interesting life."

"No, nothing interesting about me," Hanne said. "But, if you want to know something, you can feel free to ask."

I nodded, and edged closer.

"How did you get by," I asked, "while in-hiding during the war?"

"My Aunt supported us," she said. "She was an artist, and made painted plates that my Uncle would sell. My Uncle would arrange with the local farmers to bring us the wood and raw materials that she used to make decorative wood plates and paint them. We'd sit – all of us - by a large stove, and work all day, painting those bowls. The stove roared all day, but it was still always cold inside because we were on the second floor and there was always all that snow. Then, my Uncle would carry a package of these plates to the local ski resorts in the surrounding villages. This was around Innsbrook in Austria, where many tourists came to ski. They'd purchase my Aunt's bowls, so that we could make money.

"That's how we survived the war. That's how we made our money. If it hadn't been for those Nazi tourists, we wouldn't have been able to stay alive..."

CHAPTER SEVENTY-EIGHT

How did your Aunt and Uncle pick this place in Austria to live out the war? I asked.

"Well, my Aunt and Uncle were both from Prague, where their family's lived, but my Uncle saw what was coming, and made it his mission to save my family. He was German, but he really liked my Aunt's side of the family, and that was an important reason why he tried to do as much as he could.

"My Uncle's father was the chief of police in Prague, so he could use those connections to find out what was up. It actually saved my Aunt and him because the police came to him before the Gestapo. They told him that the Gestapo had discovered that his wife was Jewish, and were coming to take them away. That very night, he and my Aunt disappeared into Austria.

"My Uncle had made a plan to send me to my father's father where he thought I would be safe. Through his connections, he knew that it wouldn't be long before my mother was sent to the concentration camp. He knew that if I went with her, I probably wouldn't last long, because in the concentration camps, it was the children and the old people who were usually the first to go – transferred to other camps where no one ever came back, or were never heard from again.

"My father's father took me, but I don't think that he was very happy about it. He was on the other side. I guess that I really can't blame him, because I was putting them in danger. If the Gestapo would have found out that he was harboring me, then it would have made some serious trouble for them.

"I could tell that things were getting worse. My Uncle had left behind a contact for me – a man named Rudolf – who I was to go to if I saw that things were getting bad. So I told Rudolf, and he relayed the message to my Aunt and Uncle in Austria.

"My Aunt and Uncle took big risks in coming to get me. In those days, you couldn't travel more than ten miles from your home, or else you could be arrested. Where they were in Austria was far away from the Sudenland (where I was with my father's father). So they had to be very careful. If someone had asked for their passport on a train, it might have been it for them.

"But they came. I think that the reason why they took me was because my grandfather said that he was going to send me back to my mother. It was partly my fault. I was seven years old at the time and, like any other kid, I wanted to be with my mother. I made the mistake of telling my grandfather that, and he was saying that he was going to send me back.

"So my Aunt and Uncle came back that night, and took me away with them to Austria.

"At the time, they were living in a little town near Innsbrook called St. Jacob. They were renting from a landlady who had pretended that she was anti-Nazi. But she wasn't, and the reason why we had to leave there was my fault. I became friends with the landlady's niece. She was about my age – a little older perhaps. I suppose that I wanted someone to confide to, and, one day, I made the mistake of telling her that I was Jewish, and hiding with my Aunt and Uncle because all of my family in Prague was being taken away and sent to concentration camps. Well, they informed on us. When the Gestapo man in town came to the house, I had to say that I had lied, and made the whole thing up, and it was just that my childhood imagination had gone wild and got the best of me.

"After the interview, the Gestapo man told my Uncle that it was alright, and he wasn't going to report us, or make any further inquiries.

"Still, in the middle of a snow storm not long after, we collected all our belongings and left the village for good. My Uncle bought tickets for a city far away that would have taken days on train to get to. But really we were only on the train for two hours before we got off at a different village.

"And, the truth was, this didn't fool anyone. After the war, the Gestapo man told us that he knew exactly where we went after we left St. Jacob. But he never turned us in, and - the truth is - we could never be sure why? Maybe he was acting out of the goodness of his heart – I don't know. Hitler had already seen a number of losses by that time, and the people working for him had an idea that the war was coming to an end, and it wasn't looking good for them, and they might need something to show that they weren't completely with the Nazis – Give them an excuse to say that they weren't all bad. So, who knows? Maybe, we were the Gestapo man's excuse?..."

CHAPTER SEVENTY-NINE

"At the other village," Hanne continued, "my Uncle had arranged for us to rent a place from a farmer. It was on the second floor, and had a big stove that was always roaring. But because of all the ice and snow, it was still always cold there, and you never could get warm.

"There wasn't much to do there. When I wasn't working, I would go outside. There was really no one to talk to, and I couldn't go to school, because that would mean checking my identification, and if they found out who I really was, then it would be the end for me.

"So if anybody asked, I would say that I was fourteen and had completed my schooling. Actually, I was only ten, really. Mostly, it all seemed like a terrible nightmare that I wish I could just wake up from.

"Even after the war ended, you couldn't be sure about things. I mean, sure, we all experienced relief, but still we could never be sure that problems wouldn't start again.

A nurse entered the room and said she was tasked with helping Hanne into a gown. As the nurse assisted Hanne, April and I stepped outside.

"I can't believe it," I confided. "They were saved. They survived the Holocaust. All that oppression? How could you not be overjoyed?"

April looked out, thoughtful.

"Europe with some ruins," she said. "It was in ashes when the war was over. And the survivors had lost everything. Most lost their families. They lost their homes. They lost their possessions. They had nothing."

"Yeah, the Nazis were defeated," she continued, "but they were still in shambles. The family was gone.

"When I would talk with my grandmother about this, and tell her I wanted to go to Europe and learn about how things were, she'd tell me I live in this wonderful United States, and that we just need to be grateful, and not talk about this..."

CHAPTER EIGHTY

The nurse left the room, and April and I re-entered the room. Hanne continued her story.

"My Aunt and Uncle never did have children," she said. "My Uncle didn't want them... I think that it was because he thought that humans were on a downward phase, and the end was near for them. He was a realist, and I don't think that he had a lot of hope for humans. He was a realist, and saw things for what they were.

"To my Aunt, my Uncle was always a hero. She never uttered a bad thing about him, and worshipped the ground he walked on.

"But he felt that he really hadn't accomplished much. As well as losing all of me and my Aunt's family, he lost all of his family, too... Because after the War, when the Russians came into Czechoslovakia, the Germans living there were rounded up and sent to camps in Siberia. This is what happened to my Uncle's remaining family – his mother and his brother. Once they were taken away, they were never heard from again.

"I think that's why my Uncle came to this country – because, after everything he'd lived through, he couldn't be in Europe any longer.

"But it was never the same as before. My Aunt and Uncle had lost all their belongings. Lost all their friends. And the war took such a toll on my Uncle's health. For the rest of his life, he suffered from a heart condition that never got better. He had lots of chest pain and would have to spend days in bed... I think it was from all the times that he had to move in the cold between those villages in the mountains of Austria – finding places to sell my Aunt's plates and communicating with associates in the underground. And I'm sure that needing to take care of me didn't help, either.

"Really, I think that he was a person like everyone else. Most people don't want to see others getting hurt or mistreated. I guess that he was just a little better than most, because he acted on it..."

CHAPTER EIGHTY-ONE

I asked Hanne what became of her father?

"My father was reported as missing in action after the battle of Stalingrad," Hanne said. "Another soldier who knew my father and fought there said that when they pulled back, my father wasn't among them. He probably died there. I don't know. I never heard anything about him after that. Anyway, it was the last I ever heard of him.

"He actually got remarried during one of his last furloughs, and his wife had a son. I heard this from my grandfather. It was in the last letter that he sent me. He asked if I wanted to meet my brother? I never replied to that letter. I'm not sure why. I was pretty young at the time, and I think that I was probably confused, and maybe just wanted to cut off my relationship with that side of my family.

"I think that the marriage between my father and this woman had probably been arranged, and that side was going the other way, and I couldn't imagine that I would have had a lot in common with my brother, and, really, I didn't want to have much to do with them."

Do you remember your father?

"No," Hanne said. "I was probably 4 years old when he left, and I have no memory of him."

How did your parents meet?

"They met in music school," she said. "My father was going to be a big actor..."

Another nurse came to adjust the IV's, and April and I stepped out again.

"It's ironic," April commented. "These two German men who'd married into this Jewish family. Both had pressure to divorce their Jewish wives. Hanne's father divorced Hanne's mother, so that he could survive – And yet he wound up dying in Stalingrad. Whereas the Uncle stayed with the Aunt, and was the only surviving member of his family."

"So, love won," she concluded. "It didn't happen often, but, in this case, it did…"

CHAPTER EIGHTY-TWO

The nurse indicated that she was finished, and April and I re-entered the room.

I asked about Hanne's mother?

"My mother was a singer," she responded. "She had a very good voice. She sang for the National Conservatory. But, because of the way things were in those times, that didn't last.

"For a while she survived by giving singing lessons at home. Then, she sang in the concentration camp in Terezin. She said that that was good. The good thing about Terezin – which was probably the best of the concentration camps – was the Nazis would always show Terezin off to the concerned people who would come from neutral countries like Switzerland, or from the Red Cross.

"But just because Terezin was better than all the other camps, it still wasn't so good. You never knew when it was going to be your turn to be transported to the other camps, which were always worse, and you never heard from people again.

"Most of my family went to Terezin first before they were transported to the other camps. I tried to find out what happened to them when they were transported to the other camps, but all that information was lost and doesn't exist and I never did find out what happened to them."

I stood with my had bent, silently nodding.

"My mother survived the war," Hanne continued.

Hearing this, I looked up, surprised. I felt sure she would have perished.

"When we finally located my mother," she continued, "she was in Vienna, and we made arrangement for her to join us.

"When we met her at the train station, I could still tell that she was my mother, but she didn't look the same. She was obviously quite ill and emaciated.

"For a year, she lived with us, but it was complicated. I think that my mother understood that my Aunt and Uncle had saved my life. The children and the old people in the camps were always the first to go, and if I had been there with my mother, I wouldn't have made it.

"Still, it was difficult for my mother because I think that she also felt my Aunt and Uncle had supplanted her role with me.

"My Aunt tried to be good to my mother, and help her get over what had happened to her at the camp. But, also, there were times that my Aunt felt that my mother needed to make changes, and didn't want to baby her.

"Finally, the two of them had a big blow out, and my mother left the house and went into the village. There, she became ill, and it wasn't long before she was admitted to the hospital and died."

I looked out, unbelieving.

After all that? I thought.

Hanne excused herself to use the bathroom.

"In the family, most people think it was a suicide," April confided. "Hanne's mother's death…"

CHAPTER EIGHTY-THREE

"I don't know exactly what I felt then," Hanne continued, returning to the subject of her mother's death. "I think that I was confused. I had known so many people who had died.

"The truth is, I think that my saddest day in the whole war was in the beginning – in 1942 – when they sent grandparents to the camps.

"My grandfather had been the center of my world. He would take me on walks every day. When the family would get together, he would always take out his fiddle and play. My saddest day in the whole war was when they sent my grandparents to the camp.

"Even back then in 1942 we knew what was happening. We heard about what was going on in the concentration camps. Some of them were so terrible that you didn't believe them. People gassed. People starved. Most of this information came from the underground, so you couldn't be sure that what you heard was reliable. In the end, though, it all turned out to be true."

Yet another nurse entered the room and announced that Hanne was being discharged.

"All the blood work came back normal," the nurse said. "The doctor will call in some antibiotics to your pharmacy."

While the nurse helped Hanne dress, April and I went to the car to bring it around to the front of the hospital.

"The way Hanne and her Aunt and Uncle got to this country was they sent a letter to my grandfather, saying that they had survived the Holocaust and were in Prague and needed help to get to the United States.

"The thing was, they didn't know where my grandfather had settled," she continued. "But they remembered that he went to the

United States before the war, and they knew that he was a doctor, so what they did was write a letter and wrote on the address a lot of different cities. They wrote Washington DC, New York, L.A., and somehow somebody in the Post Office found him, and delivered the letter to my grandfather – even though Hartford, Connecticut wasn't on the letter at all.

"So my grandfather sponsored them and have them come to West Hartford. For him, they were the only ones in Europe that survived..."

Driving to Hanne's, I looked out at the ornate homes decorated with Christmas lights and other mementos of the Holiday Season, then turned to Hanne and asked how the Holocaust experience had affected her view of life?

"It makes life different," she said. "Most people, when they think about their childhood memories, I think that they have happy thoughts of the past. They go back to those thoughts when they grew older and it gives them comfort. But my thoughts are not so happy. So I don't think that I will be like a lot of those people. Instead, I take life day by day and just see what happens..."

Just before leaving the main street on the way to Hanne's home, we passed a restaurant called The Mill, where I'd heard the food was excellent.

"I have never been there," Hanne commented.

"But it's right across the way from your home," I said. "Come on, it's Christmas Eve. I'm sure it's really festive. We'll all go."

I swung the car around and turned back for the restaurant.

But the night was cold and rainy, and there were many steps to climb before the entrance.

Mike, the woman's just been released from the hospital, I thought. What are you doing exposing her to the cold and possible injury?

Then, a passing couple took an interest, and the woman offered to assist Hanne.

"I used to do this for a living," the woman said. "Here, just take my arms and will get down that last step."

Inside, the hostess seated us next to a fireplace with a view of the running waters that used to power the mill.

Hanne looked out.

"You know, I think I had been to this restaurant before," she said. "Once with my husband, Gil."

Gil had passed away only recently.

"My Aunt and Uncle disapproved of him," Hanne confided. "Because he was Puerto Rican. So, we eloped."

Really? I responded, surprised. Wouldn't think after what they'd been through, they'd hold someone's origins against anyone. How did you meet Gil?

"It was after college," Hanne said. "I was in New York working as an accountant. Gil was working as an accountant, too. He asked me if I wanted to go out with him, but I was too nervous to tell him yes. Then, his mother – who also worked in the office – told me that Gil was a good person. She was a middle aged woman, and, because of that, I thought that what she would be telling me was alright. So, the next time Gil asked me, I said yes."

Hanne paused, then smiled.

"So there," she asserted. "It was all her fault."

I laughed, and Hanne seized the moment, so that when I inquired how her marriage affected her relationship with her Aunt and Uncle, she deferred.

"It's much too nice a restaurant to continue talking about such things anymore," she insisted. "Time to talk about something else."

April agreed and engaged Hanne in a lively discussion of recent 'new arrivals' to the family and plans for future gatherings...

CHAPTER EIGHTY-FOUR

Arriving back at the house there was a letter from FQHC.

This letter is to confirm that in accordance with paragraph 13f(xix) of your employment agreement, your employment with FQHC, Inc. will be terminated effective today for failure to perform your duties to FQHC's general satisfaction...

"They did it," I said. "I can't believe it."

April stood, unaffected – Her expression offering no hint of surprise.

"You were all about giving," she said, "and the people who you were caring for were only about taking. And FQHC was just about numbers and handing out drugs and pleasing their patients, with no thought about how it was bankrupting society, and now you – Us..."

Out of work in a little room.

Where do I see myself?
I am in a little room
Feeling sorry for myself,
And the possibility that I might lose out on a career,
Because of what others might say.

April and I tried to be intimate
But I wasn't able to act.
She asked if I felt bad?
Yes.
I feel impotent.

Here I am
Sworn to love and protect her
And I was failing at that.

She was kind
And said that she hadn't done a good job of protecting me
Either.

And that's love.

If people need a physician enough
They might try me.
As was the case in Tennessee.

But this will involve more
Than ever before.

I truly do have to trust in compassion.

I have to trust in God.

And in this time
When I am questioning myself
And my ability to accept God's design
More than ever before.

ABOUT THE AUTHOR

Michael Yanuck MD PhD is a physician-scientist whose groundbreaking research at the National Institutes of Health was the basis for a FDA-approved vaccine for cancer. Following a traumatic leg injury he returned to Medicine. Intent on caring for the less fortunate, he enlisted in the National Health Service Corps, worked in urban and rural health centers throughout the country.